Essential Physiology

A guide to important principles
for nurses and laboratory technicians

Essential Physiology

Dr. D. F. Horrobin

Reader in Physiology, University of New-
castle. Formerly Professor of Medical
Physiology at the University of Nairobi.
A former fellow of Magdalen College,
Oxford.

MTP
MEDICAL AND TECHNICAL PUBLISHING CO LTD

Published by

MTP

Medical and Technical Publishing Co Ltd
St. Leonard's House, St. Leonard's Gate, Lancaster

SBN 852 000 51 0

First published 1973

Books in the 'Essential Knowledge' series for nurses:

Essential Anatomy
Essential Medicine
Essential Physics, Chemistry and Biology
**Essential Biochemistry, Endocrinology and
Nutrition**
Essential Diagnostic Tests
Essential Physiology
Essential Cardiology

PRINTED IN GREAT BRITAIN BY
EYRE & SPOTTISWOODE LTD

Contents

This series represents a new approach to medical education. Each title has been written by a leading expert who is in close touch with the education in his particular field.

These books do not cover any particular examination syllabus but each one contains more than enough information to enable the student to pass his or her examinations in that subject. The aim is rather to provide the understanding which will enable each person to get the most out of and put the most into his or her profession. Throughout we have tried to present medical science in a clear, concise and logical way. All the authors have endeavoured to ensure that students will truly understand the various concepts instead of having to memorize a mass of ill-digested facts. The message of this new series is that medicine is now moving away from the poorly understood dogmatism of not so very long ago. Many aspects of bodily function in health and disease can now be clearly and logically appreciated: what is required of the good nurse or paramedical worker is a thoughtful understanding and not a parrot-like memory.

Each volume is designed to be read in its own right. However, four titles: *Physics, Chemistry and Biology; Anatomy; Biochemistry, Endocrinology and Nutrition* and *Physiology* provide the foundations on which all the other books are based. The student who has read these four will get much more out of the other books which relate to clinical matters.

We hope that a feature of this series will be regular revision with new editions appearing about every three years. Critical comments from readers will be much appreciated as these will help us to improve later editions.

1

Introduction

Physiology is the study of the normal working of the body. It is essential that its principles should be understood by nurses and doctors, for only if you know how the body works normally can you understand what is happening during disease. This first chapter covers the whole of physiology in outline, so that as later you read the chapters devoted to giving details of the various systems, you will be able to see where each system fits into the scheme of things.

THE CELL

You can learn a great deal about physiology by considering the requirements of a simple, single-celled organism such as the amoeba. These requirements may be summarized as follows:

1. *Supplies.* All living organisms require a supply of energy if they are to survive. Plants can obtain their energy directly from the sun and by using very simple inorganic materials they can manufacture all the substances they need. But animals must obtain their energy from the complex materials which they take in as food. The energy is released by the process known as oxidation (burning), in which food is broken down and combined with oxygen to release all the energy which is required. Animals therefore obviously need a supply of food and a supply of oxygen. Since the animal body is largely made up of water, they need a supply of water as well. The amoeba finds it easy to obtain all these materials from the water which surrounds it.

2. *Waste products.* Fats and carbohydrates contain only carbon, hydrogen and oxygen. When they are oxidized, fats and carbohydrates therefore yield only carbon dioxide and water. Proteins

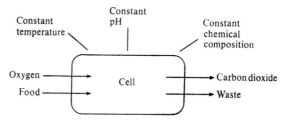

Fig.1.1 The requirements of a living cell.

in addition to carbon, oxygen and hydrogen, contain nitrogen as well. When they are broken down they give rise to ammonia as well as water and carbon dioxide. They may also lead to other more complex toxic waste products. If the cell is not to be poisoned by ammonia, by carbon dioxide or by other toxic materials these things must all be rapidly eliminated. Again in the amoeba the problem is simply solved. They are simply discharged into the surrounding water.

3. *Movement.* Animals, which cannot simply obtain their energy from light, must usually move in search of food if they are to survive. The amoeba does this by gliding along, pushing out a process of cell membrane and then sliding its cytoplasm into it.

4. *Reproduction.* Individuals are not immortal and if the species is to survive they must reproduce. The amoeba does this simply, by dividing in two.

5. *Control.* Obviously many things are happening in this apparently simple little organism the amoeba. All these separate processes must be organized and controlled so that everything works together for the good of the cell as a whole. Only now are we beginning to realize how important these control mechanisms are, even in something so simple as an amoeba.

THE HUMAN BODY

The simple solutions which the amoeba finds for its problems cannot be employed by mammals such as human beings, for two main reasons. The mammalian body is too large and it is not surrounded by water into which it can simply and safely discharge all its waste products. The human body does not consist of a single cell, but of millions upon millions of such cells. In contrast to the amoeba, each cell does not carry out the whole range of functions of which the body as a whole is capable. Instead, each cell is specialized to carry out only a small portion of the processes required for life. Specialized cells devoted to a particular function are gathered together in organs and all the organs work together so that the body as a whole can function smoothly. Nevertheless, despite this complexity, the functions of the body can still be considered under the same headings which we used for the amoeba.

1. *Supplies.* The intake of food is the function of the alimentary tract or gut. Food is taken in at the mouth and is digested in the stomach and intestines, where most of the useful material is absorbed into the body. Unusable material passes on and out in the faeces. The intake of oxygen is the function of another specialized system, the respiratory system. Air is breathed in via the nose and mouth and the oxygen from it enters the body via the lungs.

2. *Waste products.* The kidneys are specialized to excrete in the form of urine, most of the waste products produced by the body. The main exception is the gas, carbon dioxide, which is excreted via the lungs.

3. *Movement.* In order to move, a mammal requires two types of structure. First it requires a firm skeleton which will support the soft tissues and prevent them collapsing under the influence of gravity. The skeleton must not be absolutely rigid throughout and bones must be able to move in relation to one another, by being linked by joints. Second there must be a system of muscles which can pull on the bones and so move the animal.

4. *Reproduction.* In mammals reproduction is always of the sexual variety. A male produces spermatozoa which combine with the ova produced by the female. The new creature thus conceived grows in a special organ, the uterus or womb. Once the infant is born it is then nourished by milk secreted by the mammary glands. Obviously in such complex creatures as mammals, reproduction by simple division would be quite impossible.

5. *Control systems.* In any mammal, with its many organs and myriads of cells, a comprehensive system for controlling all the organs, so that they all work together for the good of the body as a whole, is clearly essential. This effective control is achieved by the operation of the nervous and hormonal (endocrine) systems.

6. *Transport between organs.* An extra problem found in large

animals, which hardly arises in the amoeba, is that of the movement of materials around the body. There must be a way in which food from the gut and oxygen from the lungs can be carried to every cell in the body. Equally, cells must be able to send carbon dioxide to the lungs and other waste products to the liver and kidneys to be destroyed and/or excreted. This linkage between the organs is the responsibility of the blood in the cardiovascular system. Blood is pumped from the heart along the arteries to every cell in the body. It then returns via the veins to the right side of the heart. From the right side of the heart it goes to the lungs and then back to the left side of the heart to be pumped out again along the arteries. By means of the blood, every single cell is put into contact with every other cell.

PHYSIOLOGICAL CONTROL MECHANISMS

The human body is so much more complex than that of the amoeba, that if it is to function satisfactorily it must have a highly organized control mechanism, consisting of the nervous and endocrine systems. There are mechanisms for controlling every aspect of the body's function and although these are often complex, they all have a number of features in common and work on much the same basic principles. In many ways they are similar to a thermostatically controlled central heating mechanism for keeping a house warm during winter. We can learn a great deal about physiological control systems by looking briefly at such a man made, relatively simple control mechanism.

Any thermostat system has three main components:

1. A thermometer which measures the temperature of the house.

2. A heating system which can raise the temperature of the house when necessary.

3. A control switch which governs the link between the thermometer and the heating system. When the thermometer indicates that the temperature in the house is too low, the control switch turns up the heating system, so bringing the house temperature up to the desired level. If on the other hand the house is too hot as indicated by the thermometer, the control switch turns the heating off and allows the temperature to fall again to the desired value.

It is obvious that the thermostat system is designed with the aim of keeping the house temperature constant in winter. Similarly the

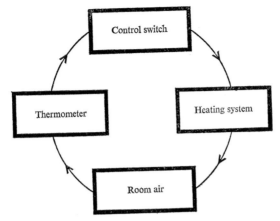

Fig.1.2. The essential elements of a household thermostat.

main aim of most of the body's control systems is to keep the properties and composition of the blood and body fluids constant. Only if the properties and composition of the blood and body fluids are kept constant in this way can all the cells function normally. The main factors which must be kept constant are:

1. *Temperature.* The rate at which chemical and biochemical reactions work depends upon the temperature. The cells in the human body are constructed to work at a constant temperature. If the blood temperature becomes too high, many reactions proceed too quickly and the functioning of many organs (especially the brain) is disturbed. The individual becomes restless and we say that he is feverish. On the other hand, if the blood temperature falls below normal, all the chemical reactions in the body go too slowly. The individual becomes lethargic and sluggish and may lose consciousness.

2. *pH.* Just as chemical reactions are affected by heat and can proceed in a controlled way only at a constant temperature, so they are affected by the acidity or alkalinity of the body fluids and can function appropriately only if the pH is kept constant. Again the functioning of many organs may be upset if the pH varies far from normal in either direction.

3. *Osmotic pressure.* Cell membranes are semi-permeable (for a full discussion of this see the book in this series on Physics, Chemistry and Biology). This means that cells must be immersed in a fluid

which has about the same osmotic pressure as the fluid inside the cells. If the osmotic pressure outside is too low, the cells will draw water inwards: they will therefore swell and may eventually burst. On the other hand, if the osmotic pressure outside is too high, water will be drawn out of the cells: they will shrink and the shrinkage may so damage the cell membrane that again the cell is destroyed.

4. *Chemical composition.* The normal behaviour of cells requires that the concentrations of many different substances in the body fluids should be kept constant. One good example is that of glucose which is used by virtually all the cells in the body and particularly by those of the brain (see book on Biochemistry, Endocrinology and Nutrition). The blood concentration of glucose must never fall too low or cells will die. Nor must it rise too high or valuable glucose will overflow into the urine and be wasted. Other vital materials whose concentration must be controlled are electrolytes such as sodium, potassium and calcium, gases such as oxygen and carbon dioxide, and innumerable other substances such as plasma proteins, thyroid hormone, the adrenal steroid hormones, parathyroid hormone and so on.

The ultimate aim therefore of most of the physiological control systems, is to maintain the constancy of the internal environment which surrounds the cells. The maintenance of this constancy is sometimes known as homeostasis.

Like the thermostat all the control mechanisms have three fundamental components:

1. They must have a way of measuring the thing which is to be controlled. In a thermostat for controlling the temperature of a house, a thermometer measures the temperature of the air inside the house. In the human body, most of the measurements are made by the parts of the nervous system which we call receptors. Perhaps the best known receptors are the eye, the ear and the ones in the skin which pick up information about touch and temperature. Each receptor is designed to collect information about some aspect of its environment: this information is then usually sent to the central nervous system (brain and spinal cord) along what are known as sensory nerves.

2. There must be a control centre which collects the information from the receptors, assesses its significance and decides what must be done. In the thermostat, this function is carried out by the switch which links the thermometer to the heating system. In the

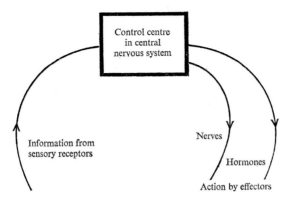

Fig.1.3. The basic components of most biological control systems.

human body, the control centre is normally to be found in the central nervous system which collects all the information from the sensory nerves.

3. There must be what are called effectors, which can alter the factor which is to be controlled. In the thermostat, the effector is the heating system which can increase the temperature of the house. In the human body there are many effectors. The control centres in the nervous system make contact with these effectors and instruct them on what to do in one of two ways, either by using nerves going from the nervous system (effector nerves) or by using hormones. Much of the rest of the book is concerned with looking in more detail at the ways in which nerves and hormones control the working of the organs in the body.

2

The nervous system

The nervous system is ultimately responsible for the control of all the other organs of the body. As such it is obviously of the greatest importance. Its construction follows the lines described at the end of the last chapter. Its most important components are:

1. *Sensory receptors.* The function of these is to collect information about the state of the body itself and also about the surrounding environment. For example, the eye and the ear gather information about the environment by using light and sound, while receptors in the skin collect information about objects coming into contact with the body. Receptors within the body itself include ones for measuring blood pressure, body temperature, blood glucose concentration, the positions of joints, the states of contraction of muscles and many other things.

2. *Sensory nerves.* The information collected by the receptors which are spread throughout the body, must be carried to the control centres in the brain and spinal cord. This is done by means of electrical changes known as nerve impulses, which are carried from the receptors to the central nervous system along sensory nerves. Sensory nerves are sometimes called afferent nerves.

3. *Central nervous system (CNS).* The central nervous system consists of the brain and the spinal cord. All the information from receptors is carried to the CNS where its significance is assessed. The CNS then makes a decision as to what action, if any, is required. The CNS can also store much of the information it receives in the form of memory.

4. *Effector nerves.* Effector nerves carry instructions from the CNS to the various organs in the body. Again these instructions are in the form of nerve impulses travelling along nerve fibres.

Effector nerves are sometimes known as motor nerves or as efferent nerves.

5. *Effector organs.* These carry out the instructions of the nervous system. The most important effectors are:

    a. Skeletal muscle. This is sometimes known as striated muscle. As its name suggests, its function is to move the skeleton.

    b. Smooth muscle. Smooth muscle is the type found in the internal organs such as the gut, the urinary tract, the walls of blood vessels and the internal genital organs.

    c. Cardiac muscle in the heart.

    d. Exocrine glands, which secrete fluids along ducts on to some body surface. Examples of exocrine glands are the pancreas and the salivary glands which secrete digestive juices, the lachrymal glands which secrete tears and the sweat glands which secrete sweat.

    e. Endocrine glands, which secrete chemicals known as hormones into the blood flowing through the gland. The hormones are then carried by the blood to all parts of the body and as will be seen later, they themselves control the behaviour of many effector organs. For example, the behaviour of important effector organs like the liver and kidney, is to a large extent determined by hormones.

NERVE CELLS

The nervous system is made up of nerve cells or neurons as they are often called. Each neuron, like almost all other cells, has a cell body containing a nucleus and cytoplasm. Neurons are however distinguished by having long fine processes arising from the cell body. Short ones which end close to the cell body are known as dendrites: they form the input end of the cell and nerve impulses arriving reach the cell by means of the dendrites. Long ones which travel some distance from the cell body are known as axons: they are the output side of the cell and nerve impulses generated by the cell leave by the axon. There are four main types of nerve cell:

    1. *CNS nerve cells.* These consist of a cell body, dendrites and an axon. The axon carries impulses from one part of the CNS to another.

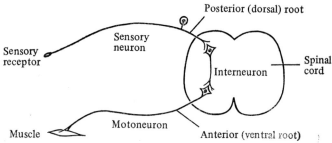

Fig.2.1. The main types of nerve cell.

2. *Somatic motoneurons.* These carry instructions from the CNS to the skeletal muscles. They consist of a cell body inside the CNS which gives rise to a very long axon. This axon leaves the CNS and carries nerve impulses to the skeletal muscles.

3. *Autonomic motoneurons.* The autonomic nervous system is concerned with controlling the behaviour of smooth muscle and of many glands throughout the body. Instructions from the CNS are carried to the effector organs not by one motoneuron, but by two in series. The axon of the first motoneuron links with the cell body of the second by means of a synapse. The synapses tend to be gathered together in groups forming structures known as the autonomic ganglia.

4. *Sensory nerve cells.* These each consist of a sense organ which gives rise to an axon. The axon carries nerve impulses to the CNS. Just before the axon reaches the CNS there is the cell body of the sensory nerve cell, usually on a short side branch.

There are two main types of nerve axon, myelinated and unmyelinated. The myelinated ones are larger in diameter and have a sheath of fatty material known as myelin: the unmyelinated ones are smaller and do not have this sheath. As far as function is concerned, the main difference between the two is that nerve impulses travel much faster along myelinated axons than along unmyelinated ones. Many of the most important tracts are therefore made up of myelinated fibres.

Links between nerve cells

The functioning of the nervous system depends on the ability of nervous impulses to jump from one nerve cell to another. The neurons are arranged so that they come into intimate contact with one another. In sensory nerves the impulses begin at the sensory receptors and travel along the axons to the CNS. There the end of each axon breaks up into minute branches which make contact with the dendrites and cell bodies of other neurons. With moto-neurons and most CNS neurons, impulses always begin at the cell bodies and travel out along the axons. The axons of CNS neurons make contact with other nerve cells. The axons of somatic moto-neurons make contact with muscle fibres. The places where two nerve fibres come into contact are known as synapses. The membranes of the two fibres do not fuse together and there is a clear gap between them filled with fluid which is outside the nerve cells and in free communication with the rest of the extra-cellular fluid in the body.

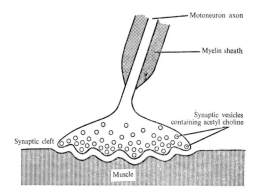

Fig.2.2. The neuromuscular junction.

The place where a motoneuron makes contact with a muscle cell is a special form of synapse, known as a neuromuscular junction: as with other synapses, there is at this junction a clear gap between the nerve cell and the muscle cell.

OUTLINE OF NERVOUS SYSTEM STRUCTURE

The nervous system consists of three main parts. Two of these, the brain within the skull and the spinal cord within the vertebral column, together form the central nervous system or CNS. The CNS is linked to most of the organs of the body by the third part, the peripheral nerves. Those peripheral nerves which are connected

directly to the brain are known as cranial nerves, while those
connected to the spinal cord are known as spinal nerves.

Like that of a worm, the body of a human being is basically
planned on a segmental basis, but by birth almost all traces of this
segmental origin have disappeared. The clearest remnants of it are
seen in the vertebral column and in the spinal cord, which lies in a
hole which runs through the vertebrae of which the column is made.
There are seven cervical vertebrae, 12 thoracic ones, 5 lumbar ones,
and 5 sacral ones fused into a single bone, the sacrum. The spinal
cord is similarly divided into segments, and corresponding to each
vertebra, a pair of nerves leaves the spinal cord. The first cervical

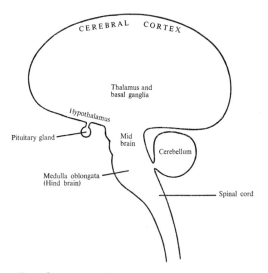

Fig.2.3. An outline of nervous system structure.

pair pass out between the first and second cervical vertebrae, the
second pair of nerves between the second and third cervical vertebrae
and so on. However, the spinal cord is actually shorter than the
hole within the vertebral column and it actually ends near the upper
lumbar region. The lower lumbar region contains no spinal cord,
but only the pairs of nerves passing obliquely down from the cord
to the appropriate holes in the vertebrae.

Each spinal nerve has two roots connecting it to the spinal cord,
one at the back (posterior) and one at the front (anterior). The

posterior root consists only of sensory fibres coming in from the sensory receptors. The anterior root consists only of motor fibres leaving the spinal cord on their way to the effector organs. Soon after leaving the spinal cord the two roots fuse and then contain a mixture of sensory and motor fibres.

As mentioned earlier, the motor system is divided into two parts, the somatic system which supplies skeletal muscles and the autonomic system which supplies smooth muscle and many glands. On the whole the somatic system is under voluntary and conscious control, while the autonomic system is not, but there are some exceptions to this rule. Structurally, the main difference between the two is that in the somatic system there is only one nerve fibre linking the CNS and the effector. In the autonomic system there are two fibres linked by a synapse. The synapses tend to be gathered together in structures known as ganglia.

The autonomic system itself is further divided into two parts, the sympathetic and the parasympathetic. The sympathetic fibres leave the thoracic and lumbar regions of the spinal cord and their ganglia lie close to the cord in a chain on either side of the vertebral column. One important ganglion, the coeliac, lies in front of the

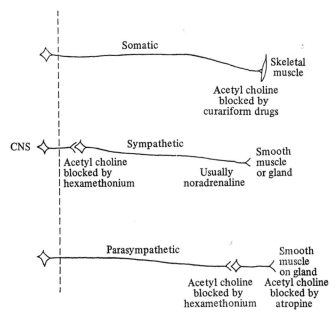

Fig.2.4. The somatic, sympathetic and parasympathetic nervous systems.

aorta at the root of the coeliac artery. In contrast, the parasympathetic nerves leave the brain and the sacral region of the
spinal cord: their ganglia are usually far from the cord in or near
the effector organs themselves.

For embryological reasons the brain is usually said to be divided
into three parts, the fore brain, the mid brain and the hind brain.
The hind brain is connected directly to the spinal cord and it consists
of the medulla oblongata and cerebellum. The medulla contains
many important control mechanisms which govern sleep, the
circulatory system and the respiratory system. The cerebellum is
essential for the control of muscular movement.

The mid brain is small but it receives much information from the
eyes and ears. It contains the structure known as the pons.

The fore brain is the largest of the three sections. It contains the
thalamus, an important sensory receiving station, the hypothalamus,
vital in the regulation of emotions and behaviour and in the control
of many body systems, and the enormous cerebral hemispheres.
The great expansion of the cerebral hemispheres is the major aspect
of nervous system structure which distinguishes man from other
animals. Many of the functional differences between man and
animals probably depend on the fore brain with its cerebral hemispheres.

Internal organization of the CNS

Within the CNS there are three main types of nervous tissue:

1. The tracts which consist of axons massed together and which
go from one part of the CNS to another.

2. Control centres for specific activities such as breathing, control
of blood pressure, control of temperature and so on.

3. The poorly understood cortex of the cerebral hemispheres,
mainly consisting of a vast mass of neurons with short axons and
which is probably responsible for such things as intelligence,
consciousness, memory and personality.

There are a few long tracts which go from the brain to the spinal
cord or vice versa, which it is important to be aware of.

A. SENSORY TRACTS. 1. Posterior columns. Sensory nerve fibres enter
the spinal cord and, turning headwards, run up the side of the cord
on which they entered. In the posterior column nuclei at the top of

the cord, they synapse with another set of nerve cells whose axons continue the tract. This tract crosses to the other side of the CNS and after synapsing again in the thalamus, eventually reaches the cerebral cortex. The posterior columns carry information about light touch and vibration.

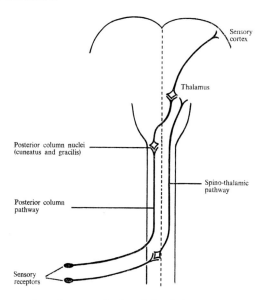

Fig.2.5. The posterior columns and spino-thalamic tracts.

2. Spino-thalamic tracts. Sensory fibres synapse immediately on entering the spinal cord. The axon of the second nerve cell in the tract then crosses to the other side of the spinal cord and runs up to the thalamus. The spino-thalamic tracts carry information about pain and temperature.

B. MOTOR TRACTS. These start in the part of the cerebral hemisphere known as the motor cortex. They cross to the opposite side on their way down through the brain and run down the opposite side of the spinal cord. In the cord they synapse with the motoneurons which leave the CNS and carry the nervous impulses to the muscles. The main motor tract is often called the pyramidal tract.

C. CEREBELLAR TRACTS. These go both up and down the spinal cord linking the cord with the cerebellum on the same side.

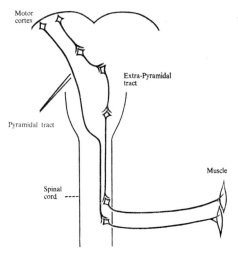

Fig.2.6. The motor tracts.

It is important to realize that almost all the important connections of the motor and sensory connections of the brain are with the opposite side of the spinal cord and of the body. The main exception is the cerebellum whose connections are with the same side of the spinal cord and body.

Cerebrospinal fluid and lumbar puncture

The brain is a hollow organ, containing spaces known as ventricles which are filled with cerebrospinal fluid. There are two lateral ventricles in the cerebral hemispheres which communicate with the third ventricle in the centre of the fore brain. This in turn communicates through the aqueduct of Sylvius with the fourth ventricle. The latter opens out on to the surface of the brain. The cerebrospinal fluid is formed by structures known as the choroid villi in the lateral and fourth ventricles. It circulates from the lateral ventricles to the fourth ventricle. Congenital or acquired blocks between the lateral ventricles and the fourth ventricle, lead to a pressure build up in the third and lateral ventricles, leading to the condition known as hydrocephalus in which the head of a fetus or infant swells because of the pressure inside the brain.

After escaping from the fourth ventricle the cerebrospinal fluid (CSF) spreads over the whole surface of the brain and spinal cord.

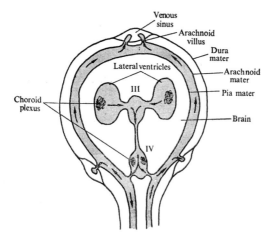

Fig.2.7. The circulation of the cerebrospinal fluid.

It circulates between the membrane known as the pia mater which covers the brain tightly and the loose, delicate membrane known as the arachnoid mater. Outside the arachnoid is the tough dura mater. There are numerous veins running within the dura mater and protrusions of the arachnoid membrane known as the arachnoid villi, stick through the dura into the veins. The CSF passes back into the blood via the arachnoid villi. In the disease known as meningitis when the membranes covering the brain become inflamed, the arachnoid villi become thickened and CSF can no longer pass through them into the blood. But the CSF is still being manufactured by the choroid plexuses and so its pressure rises well above normal levels and may interfere with brain function.

The properties of the CSF are very important in medicine. Four things matter particularly:

1. *Pressure.* This is normally about 10 to 20 cm of water. It may be raised when some disease stops the normal circulation and absorption of the CSF into the blood. The main conditions which cause a raised pressure after birth are tumours, head injuries and meningitis.

2. *Blood content.* Normally there is no blood in the CSF, but after a haemorrhage in some part of the brain, the CSF may become blood-stained.

3. *Glucose content.* Normally the glucose concentration is 50–80

mg/100 ml. However in meningitis, bacteria may use up the glucose and its concentration may be much lower than normal.

4. *Protein content.* This is normally very low indeed but it may be raised in meningitis or in the presence of a cerebral tumour. CSF is normally a watery and crystal clear fluid. After a haemorrhage in the brain it may be reddish or yellowish, but still clear. In meningitis it is often cloudy.

Clearly it is important for a doctor to be able to sample the CSF reasonably easily. This is usually done by performing a lumbar puncture, and is made possible by the fact that the spinal cord is considerably shorter than the vertebral column and the sac of dura mater and arachnoid mater within that column. There is

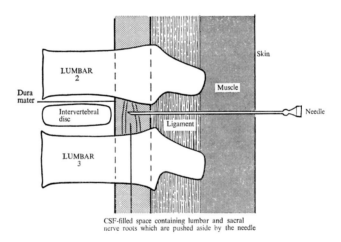

CSF-filled space containing lumbar and sacral
nerve roots which are pushed aside by the needle

Fig.2.8. The principle of the lumbar puncture.

therefore a fluid filled space in the lumbar region of the spine below the end of the cord. Under local anaesthetic a long needle is pushed between the lumbar vertebrae (usually 2 and 3) in the mid-line. When the needle enters the CSF filled space, the pressure of the fluid can be measured and a sample withdrawn.

THE NERVOUS IMPULSE

The functioning of the nervous system depends upon the electrical disturbances known as nerve impulses (or sometimes as action potentials) which travel along axons, carrying messages from one part of the nervous system to another. It is possible to detect a nerve impulse by means of an electrode pushed into an axon and connected to a delicate electrical recording instrument. This demonstrates that when the nerve axon (or fibre) is resting and no impulses are passing along it, the inside of the fibre is electrically negative to the surrounding fluid. The difference is about 70 millivolts (1 millivolt is 1 thousandth of a volt). Nerve impulses can be started

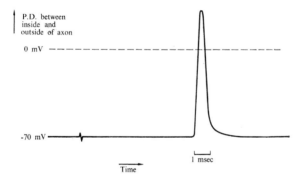

Fig.2.9. An action potential.

in axons in a number of ways, one of which is to give an electric shock to the nerve. Suppose we started off by giving the nerve a very small shock followed by a series of shocks of gradually increasing size. The small shocks would have no effect. Once a certain critical shock strength had been reached (known as the threshold value)

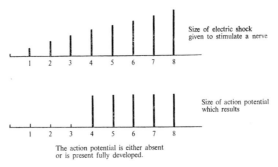

Fig.2.10. The all-or-nothing principle.

an impulse would be fired off. The recording electrode would reveal that during the impulse the inside of the fibre momentarily becomes positive to the outside and then within about a thousandth of a second returns to its resting value. If shocks which are bigger than the threshold value are given, they also produce impulses but the impulses are of exactly the same size as the first one. Bigger shocks do not produce bigger impulses. An impulse is either not there at

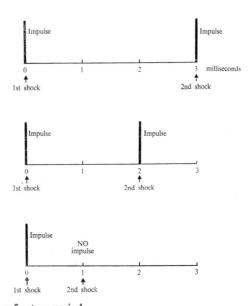

Fig.2.11. The refractory period.

all, or it is there in its fully-developed form: there is no half-way stage. This is therefore known as an all-or-nothing phenomenon.

If two shocks are given to the nerve, one after the other, two action potentials are produced unless the second shock follows the first within one thousandth of a second or so. If the second shock follows the first after such a short time interval it fails to produce a second impulse. During the action potential and immediately afterwards, the nerve is unresponsive to stimulation. The period when the nerve is unresponsive is known as the refractory period.

Calcium and tetany

Normally impulses do not begin in nerve cells spontaneously. They are fired off either by sensory receptors or by an impulse from another nerve cell arriving at a synapse. In the resting state no impulses are fired off, because the resting nerve membrane normally has a stable potential difference across it and this potential does not vary spontaneously. However, the stability of the nerve membrane seems to depend on the presence of precisely the right concentration of calcium ions in the blood and body fluids. The calcium is found in two main forms, as free calcium ions and as calcium bound to proteins in the plasma. The two interact with one another as follows:

$$\text{Calcium ions} + \text{protein} \rightleftharpoons \text{Calcium-protein}$$

It is only the free calcium ions on the left hand side of the equation which are physiologically active in maintaining the stability of nerve membranes. If the concentration of free calcium ions falls too low, nerve axons become unstable and start to fire off many impulses spontaneously. The impulses which arise in motor nerves go to muscles and cause involuntary twitches and spasms. These twitches are particularly evident in the muscles on the inner side of the hand and forearm and when severe they give rise to a typical hand position: this is often known as 'accoucheur's hand', because it is similar to the hand position used by a midwife when carrying out a vaginal examination. The facial muscles also often twitch and may sometimes be thrown into spasm if the cheek is tapped where it overlies the facial nerve (Chvostek's sign). The impulses fired off in sensory axons produce tingling sensations. The combination of tingling and muscle twitches is known as tetany and is always caused by a low concentration of free calcium ions in the blood.

Tetany is sometimes caused by a low total calcium concentration, i.e. both the protein-bound and free ionic forms are reduced in amount. This may occur during disease of the parathyroid glands if the output of parathyroid hormone is low. However this is a rare form of tetany. Much more common is the situation in which the total amount of calcium in the blood is normal but the concentration of calcium ions is low because they have been bound by protein. Thus more calcium than usual is in the protein-bound form and less is in the form of calcium ions. This commonly occurs if the blood becomes too alkaline, because alkalinity causes the protein to bind the calcium. Alkalinity may sometimes be caused by excessive vomiting of acid gastric juice. Much more frequently it is caused by overbreathing. If you breathe too hard, carbon dioxide is removed more quickly than usual by the lungs and its concentration in the blood falls. Since the acidity of the blood depends to a large extent on carbon dioxide, the fall in carbon dioxide level means an increase in alkalinity. This means that free calcium ions become bound to protein and tetany results. This situation occurs frequently in hysterical and over-excited individuals and also in childbirth. The cure is simple. A bag should be put over the face for a short while so that the patient breathes back the carbon dioxide he or she has just breathed out. This quickly brings the blood carbon dioxide level back to normal, the alkalinity decreases, calcium ions are released from the protein and the tetany vanishes.

Neuromuscular and synaptic transmission

Impulses jump from one nerve cell to another, or from a nerve cell to an effector organ or gland such as a muscle or gland, by a process of chemical transmission. In this process, when an impulse reaches the end of an axon it causes the release of a chemical which is stored in the fine branches at the end of the axon. The chemical enters the gap between the axon and the next nerve cell, muscle or gland. It crosses the gap and becomes attached to the membrane of the nerve cell, muscle or gland. When it becomes attached, it fires off another nerve impulse or it makes the effector operate.

The process is best understood in the case of the link between a motoneuron and the skeletal muscle fibre which it supplies. This link is often known as the neuromuscular junction. The motoneuron releases a chemical known as acetyl choline which becomes attached to the muscle fibre membrane and sets up an impulse there. Almost as soon as this has happened, the acetyl choline is destroyed by an enzyme known as cholinesterase which is found at the neuro-

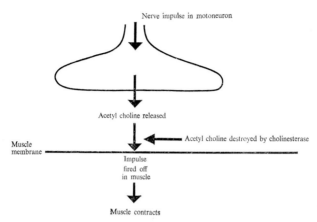

Nerve impulse in motoneuron

Acetyl choline released

Muscle membrane

Acetyl choline destroyed by cholinesterase

Impulse fired off in muscle

Muscle contracts

Fig.2.12. The working of the neuromuscular junction.

muscular junction. This destruction allows the muscle membrane to return to its resting state, ready for another nerve impulse. A number of important drugs alter the behaviour of the neuromuscular junction:

1. Drugs which paralyse the muscle. These are of two sorts:

   a. Curariform drugs such as tubocurarine. This group of drugs was originally derived from a South American arrow poison which was used to paralyse hunted animals. Curare is similar enough to acetyl choline to become attached to the muscle membrane, but it cannot stimulate the membrane or be destroyed by cholinesterase. It therefore prevents acetyl choline reaching the muscle. If the acetyl choline cannot reach the muscle it cannot stimulate the muscle to contract and so the muscle is paralysed.

   b. Drugs such as succinyl choline (Scoline). These drugs are also similar to acetyl choline and become attached to the muscle membrane. They are even similar enough to stimulate the membrane and to cause a contraction. But they cannot be destroyed by cholinesterase and so they remain attached to the muscle and prevent it returning to its resting state ready for another impulse. This means that they first produce a twitch and then paralyse the muscle because they cannot be removed. Every nurse who has ever watched an anaesthetist intubate a patient has seen the characteristic action of these

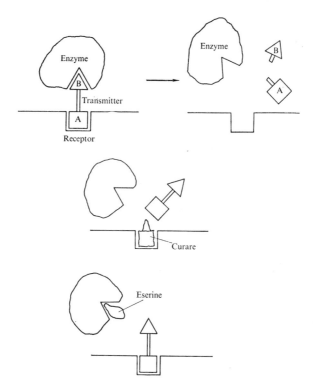

Fig.2.13. Schematic diagram of the action and destruction of acetyl choline and of the modes of action of curare and eserine. The A part of the acetyl choline molecule fits into the muscle receptor while the B part can become attached to the enzyme cholinesterase.

drugs, which on intravenous injection produce first a series of muscle twitches and then paralysis.

2. Drugs which block the action of the enzyme cholinesterase (e.g. eserine, neostigmine, prostigmine). In the presence of these drugs acetyl choline is not destroyed in the usual way and so can act for a longer period. To some extent these drugs can reverse the action of the muscle relaxant drugs described in 1. They are also used in the disease myasthenia gravis. In this disease the patient behaves as though his motor nerves do not release enough acetyl choline to stimulate the muscle properly. By giving anti-cholinesterase drugs, the action of the acetyl choline that is released can be more prolonged and effective, and muscle power may increase thus enabling the patient to live a relatively normal life.

Synaptic transmission in the ganglia of the autonomic nervous system is also quite well understood. At all autonomic ganglia, the chemical transmitter between the two nerve cells is acetyl choline. Transmission at the ganglia can be interfered with by a group of drugs similar to those which block transmission at the neuromuscular junction. They are known as the ganglion-blocking agents and interfere with all actions of the autonomic nervous system. In the parasympathetic system, the nerve cells which go from the ganglia to the effectors also release acetyl choline. The action of the acetyl choline at the receptors may be blocked by means of a widely used drug known as atropine. Atropine is used in anaesthesia, because in response to many anaesthetics the parasympathetic nerves which

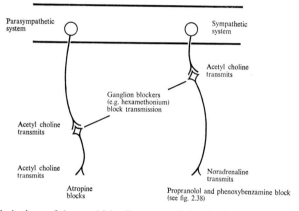

Fig.2.14. Actions of drugs which affect transmission in the autonomic NS.

supply the bronchi, stimulate the glands there to pour out large amounts of sticky secretion. This narrows the lung tubes and may predispose to the development of pneumonia later. Atropine is therefore often given some time before an anaesthetic in order to block the actions of these nerves and to prevent the excessive production of secretions.

The nerves which travel from sympathetic ganglia to effectors almost all release a substance known as noradrenaline (norepinephrine). The main exceptions to this rule are the sympathetic nerves which go to the sweat glands and which release acetyl choline.

In the CNS chemical transmission is as yet not so well understood and none of the chemical transmitters involved has as yet been identified. One thing about the CNS is clear, and that is that it is very complex. As well as transmitters which stimulate cells to fire off impulses, there are inhibitory chemicals which prevent nerve cells from firing.

SKELETAL MUSCLES

There are three main types of muscle, skeletal or striated, smooth or unstriated and cardiac. The first two will be discussed in this chapter, while cardiac muscle will be considered in the chapter on the heart.

Skeletal muscle is so-called because it moves the skeleton. It forms the bulk of the soft tissue in the limbs and in the walls of the chest and abdomen. Each bulky muscle is made up of a very large number of long thin cells known as muscle fibres. Under the microscope these cells can be seen to have very fine cross stripes, hence the name striated muscle. The striations are there because of the precise and orderly arrangement within the muscle fibre, of the tiny protein fibrils which bring about contraction.

Each muscle fibre is supplied by a nerve fibre which is a branch of a motoneuron axon. All motoneurons split up into several branches and supply several muscle fibres. One motoneuron, its branches and the muscle fibres it supplies, are all together known as a motor unit. In coarse muscles, such as those of the leg, where delicate movements

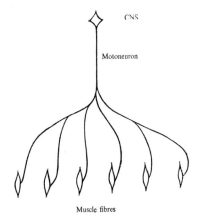

CNS

Motoneuron

Muscle fibres

Fig.2.15. A motor unit.

are not required, the motor units are large: a single motoneuron may split up to supply 200 or more muscle fibres. In contrast, in small muscles which carry out fine movements such as those of the fingers or eyes, the motor units are very small and may contain only five or six muscle fibres: this gives the nervous system the ability to control movements much more precisely.

A muscle fibre may be regarded as a nerve axon with a contraction mechanism wrapped up inside it. When the muscle is stimulated either by acetyl choline released from a nerve or by an artificial electric shock, a nerve-like impulse quickly spreads over the muscle fibre membrane. As in nerves, the impulse is over within not much more than 1/1000th of a second and the muscle is then ready to conduct another impulse. Within the muscle fibre is the contractile mechanism made up primarily of the proteins actin and myosin. As the impulse spreads over the fibre it stimulates these proteins to contract and the muscle fibre shortens. It reaches its shortest length within 20–50 milliseconds (one millisecond is 1/1000th of a second) and relaxes over 50–300 milliseconds. This means that the whole contraction process following a single nerve impulse is over within less than half a second.

The impulse which spreads over a muscle fibre is followed, like a nerve impulse, by a refractory period which lasts for about 1 millisecond. Unlike the impulse, the contraction process which the impulse triggers off has no refractory period. This means that if a second impulse arrives before the first contraction is over, the second

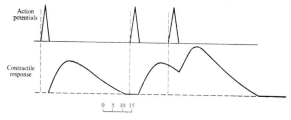

Fig.2.16a. Diagram to show how two action potentials which are close together can produce a larger muscle contraction. Scale is in milliseconds.

contraction will add on to the first. This can occur because the refractory period following the impulse is so short and, even allowing for the refractory state, it is possible for the muscle fibre to

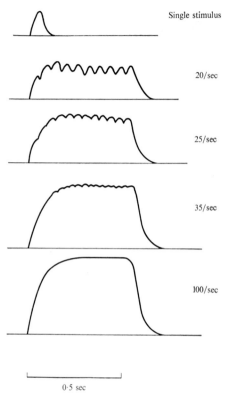

Fig.2.16b. Diagram to show the effects of different rates of nerve stimulation on muscle contraction. The response becomes a completely smooth tetanus at stimulation frequences above 50/sec.

conduct an impulse about every two milliseconds. Since the contraction process takes several hundred milliseconds in all, it is obvious that many impulses may travel over the muscle fibre before the contraction which resulted from the first impulse of a series is completed. If a series of impulses follow one another at intervals of less than about 100 milliseconds, there is no time for complete relaxation between each one and the next, and the result is a wavy contraction known as incomplete tetanus. If impulses follow one another with less than 20–40 milliseconds between them, there is no time for any relaxation whatever and the result is a smooth, sustained contraction which is known as a complete tetanus (note that tetanus and tetany are two different words with quite different meanings: note also that tetanus when it refers to muscle contraction has a different meaning from when it refers to the disease). The smooth contractions of muscles which occur in normal conditions are due to rapid trains of impulses which bring about a tetanus.

SMOOTH MUSCLE

Smooth muscle is very important in the body. It is the type of muscle which is found in blood vessels, in the gut, in the lungs, in the ureters and bladder and in the internal genital organs. The fibres themselves are much smaller than skeletal muscle fibres and they do not show striations. They contain actin and myosin and the fundamental mechanism of contraction may be the same in both skeletal and smooth muscle. However, in smooth muscle the contractions appear to be much less efficiently organized and contractions are slow to develop and to relax. However, in most of the situations in which smooth muscle is found, such relatively slow contractions are just what is required.

Many smooth muscle fibres also differ from skeletal muscle fibres in that they can contract spontaneously in the absence of nervous impulses. Simple stretch often makes a smooth muscle fibre contract. However, smooth muscles do receive nerve fibres which may release acetyl choline (parasympathetic fibres) or noradrenaline sometimes called norepinephrine (sympathetic fibres). Smooth muscles are also affected by circulating adrenaline (epinephrine) released from the adrenal medulla. In general, acetyl choline and noradrenaline both tend to cause smooth muscle contraction. Adrenaline sometimes causes contraction and sometimes relaxation, for reasons which will be explained in the section on the autonomic nervous system and the adrenal medulla.

SENSE ORGANS

The function of sense organs is to supply the CNS with information about the external environment and also about things which are happening inside the body (the internal environment). Sense organs (or receptors as they are called) which monitor the internal environment are known as proprioceptors. Normally we are not consciously aware of the fact that they are functioning: there are exceptions to this rule, such as the sense organs, which provide information about the state of the bladder. Sense organs which monitor the external environment are sometimes known as exteroceptors and we are usually consciously aware of what they are doing.

The most important exteroceptors are:

1. Sense organs in the skin, which detect touch, pressure, cold and heat.

2. Taste receptors, especially on the tongue, which monitor the chemical composition of the food. There appear to be four main types for sour, sweet, bitter and metallic tastes.

3. Smell receptors in the nasal passages, which monitor the chemical composition of the air. There may be seven different types. The senses of smell and taste are very closely linked. For example, many foods 'taste' quite different when our sense of smell is defective as a result of a bad cold. This shows that the sensation which we usually call 'taste' depends on both taste and smell receptors.

4. The eyes and ears, which enable us to learn about what is happening at some distance away from the body. These senses will be discussed more fully later in this chapter.

Proprioceptors

These are vital for the minute by minute regulating processes which keep our bodies running normally and about which we are not usually aware. Some of the more important proprioceptors are:

1. Receptors which measure the blood pressure (baroreceptors). These are found in the walls of many arteries but particularly in the aorta and in the carotid sinus where the internal and external carotid arteries divide.

2. Receptors which monitor the chemical composition of the blood. There are very many different types. Important ones are oxygen receptors in the carotid body, pH receptors in the carotid body, carbon dioxide receptors in the brain and carotid body, glucose receptors in the pancreas and the brain and receptors for many different hormones, usually in the brain.

3. Receptors which measure the osmotic pressure of the blood. When an animal loses water, the osmotic pressure of its blood may rise; when it gains water the osmotic pressure of the blood may fall. Receptors in the part of the brain called the hypothalamus measure blood osmotic pressure.

4. Receptors in the hypothalamus which measure the temperature of the blood.

5. Receptors in the gut which measure how much it is being stretched by the gut contents and which monitor the chemical composition of the contents.

6. Receptors which monitor the state of the locomotor system. Joint receptors monitor the positions of joints while Golgi organs in the muscle tendons and muscle spindles among the muscle fibres, measure the degree of relaxation or contraction of a muscle.

This is by no means a complete list of all the proprioceptors in the body, but it does include the most important ones.

The ear

Sound travels through air because the air molecules are set vibrating by the source of the sound. This is most obvious when the sound is generated by a vibrating string as in a guitar, but it applies to all types of sound. The ear is a specialized device for picking up these vibrations and for transforming them into nervous impulses. The ear consists of three main parts:

1. *The outer ear.* This comprises the pinna and a tube leading into the side of the skull known as the external auditory meatus. In animals the pinna may be used for collecting sound waves, but in human beings it seems to have lost this function. The meatus contains ceruminous glands which produce wax. The human race seems to be genetically divided into two types: in one the wax is hard and flaky and it falls out easily causing no trouble: in the other the wax is sticky and often blocks the meatus. Accumulation of wax is a common cause of curable deafness.

2. *The middle ear.* This consists of the ear drum, or tympanic membrane and the three bony ossicles known as the incus, malleus and stapes. The stapes is shaped like a stirrup and its foot piece fits tightly into the oval window between the middle ear and inner ear. The actual sound-detecting mechanism is in the inner ear which is a fluid-filled chamber. The problem which must be solved by the middle ear, is to transfer the sound vibrations from the air to the inner ear fluid. Normally sound moves from air to water very inefficiently. The air is much lighter than the water and the air vibrations simply bounce off the surface of the water without setting

the water molecules vibrating. The middle ear gets around this problem in two ways:

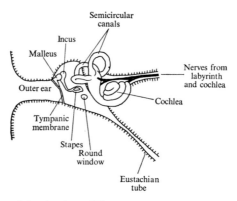

Fig.2.17. Outline of the structure of the ear.

a. The tympanic membrane which closes off the middle ear from the outer ear is set vibrating by sound. The three bony ossicles transfer these vibrations to the oval window. The tympanic membrane is about fifteen times greater in area than the oval window and so all the energy of the vibrations of the ear drum is concentrated on the window. The effect is rather like that of a drawing pin: it is easy to push a drawing pin into a notice board because all the force which is applied to the broad head of the pin can be concentrated on the tiny point. Thus the vibrations of the oval window are much more forceful than those of the much larger tympanic membrane and are able to set the inner ear fluid vibrating.

b. The ossicles are so arranged that the movements of the stapes at the round window are only about $\frac{3}{4}$ of those of the head of the malleus at the ear drum. In such a linked chain of bones, the product of the distance moved and the force of the move-ment must be the same at the beginning and the end of the chain. If the stapes moves only $\frac{3}{4}$ of the distance moved by the malleus with each vibration, then the force of movement of the stapes must be 4/3 times that of the malleus.

Because of these two mechanisms, the force of movement of the oval window is about twenty times that of the movement of the ear drum and this enables the vibrations of the air to set the fluid in the inner ear vibrating as well. If you have difficulty in understanding this, think about the drawing pin analogy for a while. If you push the flat head of a drawing pin which has lost its point against a cork notice board, you will make little impression. But a normal drawing pin penetrates the cork easily because the force which you apply to the whole head is concentrated on the point which can easily penetrate the cork.

3. *The inner ear.* This is the place where sound is actually converted into nervous impulses. The organ where this process occurs is

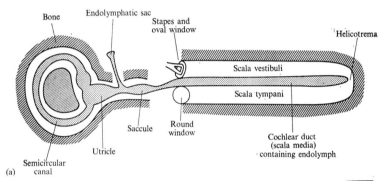

Fig.2.18*a*. Schematic outline of the inner ear: for purposes of clarity the cochlea has been uncoiled.

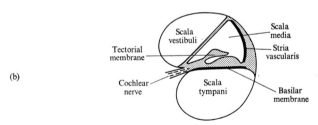

Fig.2.18*b*. Transverse section of the cochlea.

known as the cochlea and is shown schematically in Fig.2.18. There are two outer tubes enclosed by bone known as the scala vestibuli and the scala tympani, which communicate with one another at the apex of the cochlea. Between these two is a membranous tube known as the scala media which contains the basilar membrane and the organ of Corti. The three tubes are coiled around like a snail shell, but in the diagram for simplicity's sake they are shown as though they were straightened out. The hole from the scala vestibuli to the middle ear is closed by the stapes in the oval window while the scala tympani is closed by the membrane across the round window. During vibrations, as the oval window is pushed in by the stapes the round window is pushed out and vice versa. The resulting vibrations in the fluid set the basilar membrane vibrating. Low pitched sounds cause the whole membrane to vibrate. As sounds become higher, only part of the membrane vibrates until with the highest sounds only a small length of basilar membrane right next to the oval window is moving.

A simplified diagram of the organ of Corti is shown in Fig.2.19. The basilar membrane carries cells which have hairs sticking out from their upper surfaces. These hairs are embedded in the tectorial membrane. When the basilar membrane vibrates, the tectorial membrane slides over it, pulling on the hairs. This pulling fires off impulses in the nerves which supply the hair cells. Each hair cell has its own nerve fibre. Therefore the brain, by seeing which nerve fibres are firing the most impulses, can tell which part of the basilar

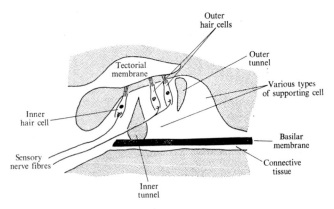

Fig.2.19. The organ of Corti.

membrane is vibrating most: since the part of the membrane which vibrates the most depends on the pitch of the sound, the brain can identify what the pitch is. The loudness of the sound depends on just how active the nerve with most activity is.

DEAFNESS. There are essentially two types of deafness, usually known as nerve and conduction deafness. In conduction deafness, the mechanism for conducting the sound to the inner ear via the external auditory meatus, the tympanic membrane, the ossicles and the oval window is defective. The commonest causes of conduction deafness are wax in the outer ear and damage to the ear drum following a middle ear infection. With conduction deafness, sound can still travel to the inner ear via vibrations in the bones of the skull: this is much less effective than the normal mechanism, but such patients can be greatly helped by amplification of the sounds by the use of a hearing aid.

With nerve deafness, on the other hand, either the cochlea or the auditory nerve itself is damaged. This means that even if sound conduction to the inner ear is normal, there will be defective hearing. If the auditory nerves are completely destroyed, no hearing aid can help. Overdoses of drugs such as streptomycin and some of the newer antibiotics are not uncommon causes of nerve deafness because they seem to damage the auditory nerve fibres.

THE EAR AND BALANCE. The ear is not only the organ of hearing, it is also the organ of balance. The part of the ear concerned with balance is known as the labyrinth and the nerve which supplies it is the vestibular nerve. The labyrinth contains the semi-circular canals which inform the brain whenever the head is rotated. On each side there are three linked semi-circular tubes filled with fluid. Each of the three has at one point a dilatation known as the ampulla. Projecting into the ampulla is a structure rather like a swing door known as the crista. The crista has a rich nerve supply. When the head rotates, the walls of the canals move with the skull, but initially the fluid within the tubes (the endolymph) tends to get left behind: this fluid therefore pushes on the crista, bending it over and firing off a series of nerve impulses. The rate and direction of head movement can be determined by the brain noting which of the canals is generating the most impulses and just how fast the impulses are being fired.

Other parts of the labyrinth are the utricle and saccule. These provide information about the position of the head when it is stationary and also about acceleration. Essentially these organs consist of blobs of chalk mounted on stiff hairs which are in turn connected to nerve fibres. When the head is accelerated, the hairs bend backwards, the degree of bending depending on the speed

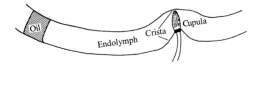

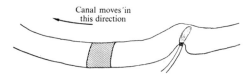

Fig.2.20. The response to rotation of the crista of a semi-circular canal. The oil droplet injected into the canal shows that the movement of the fluid lags behind the movement of the canal wall.

of the acceleration. When the head is tilted, the hairs also bend and the impulse activity in the nerves increases in proportion to the degree of bending. By assessing this activity the brain can know the position of the head.

The eye

Vision can roughly be split up into three separate processes. First, there is a focussing system at the front of the eye consisting of the lens and the cornea. The function of these elements is to produce a sharp image on the retina at the back of the eyeball. Secondly, the retina converts this sharp image into a pattern of nervous impulses. Thirdly these impulses are transmitted to the occipital part of the brain at the back of the head and it is with this part of the brain that we actually 'see'.

STRUCTURE. The structure of the eye is shown in Fig.2.21. The eye is divided into two compartments by the ciliary body and the lens. The posterior compartment is filled with jelly-like vitreous humour, while the anterior compartment is filled with watery aqueous humour. The anterior compartment is further sub-divided into anterior and posterior chambers. The posterior chamber is the small space between the lens and the iris, while the anterior chamber is the slightly larger space in front of the iris. The aqueous humour is

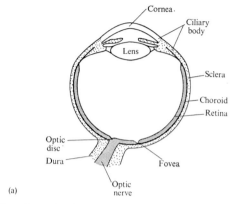

(a)

Fig.2.21a. Outline of eye structure.

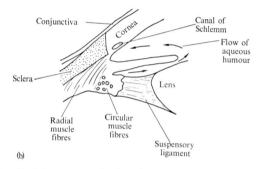

(b)

Fig.2.21b. Detail of the corneo-scleral angle.

secreted by the blood vessels of the anterior surface of the ciliary body and of the iris. It passes forwards through the hole in the iris known as the pupil and escapes into the canal of Schlemm. The pressure of the aqueous humour is normally about 15 mm Hg but if for any reason drainage into the canal is blocked, the pressure rises. This situation is called glaucoma. It causes intense pain and unless the pressure is quickly brought down the retina may be permanently damaged. There are three basic ways of reducing the pressure:

1. Drugs which constrict the pupil pull the iris tissue away from the canal and allow freer drainage of the fluid.

2. Drugs which reduce the rate of formation of the aqueous humour, such as acetazoleamide ('Diamox').

3. Surgical methods of making a tiny hole in the eyeball and so allowing the fluid to drain away.

FOCUSSING. The focussing system consists of two main elements, the cornea and the lens. The cornea is the more important. This is shown by the fact that when the lens becomes opaque in old age or because of disease (cataract), it can be removed. The person is then able to see reasonably well with the aid of glasses. However, the cornea is a fixed lens: it cannot alter its focussing power depending on how far away is the object to be viewed. The adjustable focussing of the eye depends on the lens. The cornea roughly focusses the image so that it falls just behind the retina. The final fine focussing on the retina is done by varying the power of the lens. In healthy young people the lens is able to adjust, so that both far distant objects and ones a few inches in front of the nose can be brought into sharp focus. With ageing, the focussing power of the lens is reduced and while distant objects can usually be seen normally, ones close to the face cannot be brought into focus. Thus older people almost always require glasses for reading.

The adjustments of the lens depend on the ciliary muscles. The lens itself is in some ways rather like an elastic ball, which tends to assume a spherical shape when removed from the body. When in

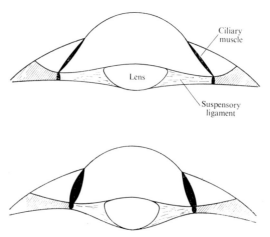

Fig.2.22. The control of the ciliary muscle during focussing. In the upper figure the muscle is relaxed and the suspensory ligament is taut, flattening the lens. In the lower figure the contracted muscle takes the tension off the suspensory ligament and allows the lens to become more globular.

the body, there is attached around its margin the tough suspensory ligament which slings the lens from the ciliary body and permanently keeps it partially flattened and less globular than it would normally be. The flatter the lens the weaker it is: the more globular it is the more powerful it is. When the ciliary muscles contract they pull the suspensory ligaments inward. This takes tension off the lens and allows it to become more globular and powerful. When the ciliary muscles relax, the suspensory ligaments flatten the lens making it weaker. When we are looking at near objects, the light rays need to be bent more than when we are looking at distant objects. Therefore when looking at things close to the eye, the lens must be more globular and the ciliary muscles must be working.

In normal people, when the ciliary muscles are relaxed and the lens is flattened, distant objects are in perfect focus. However, if we want to look at an object nearer than about 20 feet away, the lens must become more powerful and the ciliary muscles must contract in order to allow it to become more globular. The changes in the eyes which occur when one looks at a nearby object after looking at a distant one are known as accommodation. Accommodation consists of three processes:

1. The contraction of the ciliary muscles to make the lens more powerful.

2. The muscles of the eyeball act to make the eyes look towards the mid-line. This is known as convergence.

3. The pupils become smaller, so covering up the outermost parts of the lens. This is because the central part of the lens focusses much more accurately than the outer parts. When the light rays must be bent considerably in order to achieve focussing, the image is much sharper if only the central part of the lens is used.

The front surface of the cornea must be continually kept moist if it is not to be damaged. This is achieved partly by the tears and partly by oily secretions from glands in the eyelids. Tears are secreted by the lacrymal glands at the lateral edges of the eye sockets. They flow across the eyeball and drain into the nasal passages via the lacrimal duct at the medial side of the eye socket. Tears contain lysozyme, an enzyme which can kill some bacteria. The rate of secretion of tears is increased by stimuli which could potentially damage the eyes such as poisonous gases or dust. It is also increased by emotion.

FOCUSSING DEFECTS. Normal vision in young people is known as emmetropia. If the eyeball is too short or if the cornea and lens are too powerful, distant objects are focussed in front of the eyeball and are always blurred: since there is no way of reducing the power of the focussing system they can never be brought into sharp focus. This condition is known as myopia. Because of the power of their system, people with myopia (short sight) can see objects which are very close to their eyes, almost literally at the ends of their noses.

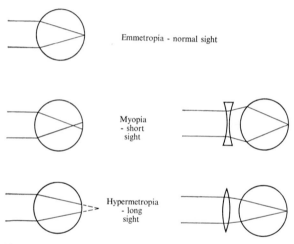

Emmetropia - normal sight

Myopia - short sight

Hypermetropia - long sight

Fig.2.23. Short and long sight and their correction by spectacles.

The opposite defect to myopia is known as hypermetropia or long sight. Either the eye is too short or the focussing system is too weak and even distant objects tend to be focussed behind the retina. By accommodation which increases the power of the lens, distant objects can be brought into focus but near ones can never be seen sharply.

Fortunately both short and long sight can easily be corrected by the use of appropriate spectacles. With myopia the overall power of the focussing system must be made less and so a diverging (concave) lens must be put in front of the eye. With hypermetropia the overall power of the focussing system must be increased and so a converging (convex) lens is placed in front of the eyes.

The third common focussing defect is known as astigmatism. In this condition the focussing power of the lens system (usually of

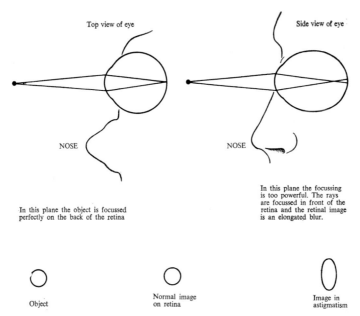

Fig.2.24. Astigmatism.

the cornea) is different in different planes. As a result, rays falling in, say, the vertical plane may be focussed precisely on the retina, while those falling in the horizontal plane are focussed in front or behind. As a result, round objects tend to appear oval.

IRIS. The iris has two main functions. First it constricts in bright light and opens up in darkness. This helps to control the amount of light which falls on the retina. In bright light the iris cuts down the amount of light, while in dim light it opens up as widely as possible in order to let in as much light as possible.

The second function of the iris is to cover up the outer parts of the lens whenever the light is bright enough to permit this. Like all lenses, the focussing of the lens of the human eye tends to be inaccurate when light falls on its edges. The lens functions best when light is passing through its centre. The iris thus helps to ensure that the light falls in the best part of the lens.

THE RETINA. The retina is the part of the eye which is sensitive to light and which converts the image into a pattern of nervous impulses.

The retina contains two types of light receptors, the rods and the cones. The rods are not sensitive to colour but they can pick up very dim light and it is they which function at night. The cones can detect colours but they are much less sensitive than the rods and so function only when the light is relatively bright.

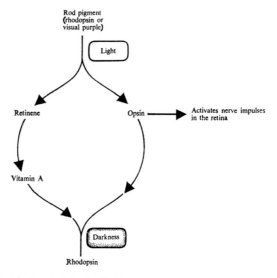

Fig.2.25. The biochemical basis of vision.

Both rods and cones contain pigments which are broken up when light falls upon them. The substances produced by this breakdown can then generate nervous impulses. The pigment that is found in the rods is known as visual purple or rhodopsin. Vitamin A is essential for the manufacture of visual purple. In the absence of the vitamin no visual purple can be manufactured and so vision in dim light at night is defective: this is known as 'night blindness'.

The retina has two further layers of cells in addition to the rods and cones. The rods and cones send their impulses to the bipolar cells and the bipolar cells send impulses to the ganglion cells. The axons of the ganglion cells then leave the eyeball via the optic nerve and go to the brain. Paradoxically the rods and cones are on the outermost layer of the retina and so light has to pass through the other cells before it reaches the light sensitive receptors. Only in

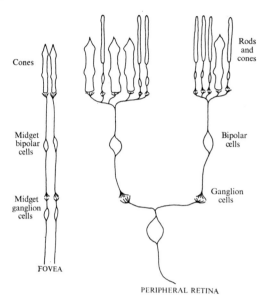

Fig.2.26. The structure of the retina. At the fovea each cone has a 'private line' in the optic nerve. In the outer part of the retina several rods and cones may share the same line.

one area of the retina is this not true. This is the fovea which contains no rods but only cones. In the fovea the ganglion and bipolar cells are pushed to one side so that light can fall directly on the cones. Visual acuity is highest when the image falls on the fovea and so when you look at an object the eyes automatically move so that the

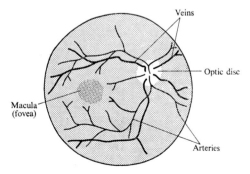

Fig.2.27. The retina as seen through an ophthalmoscope. The optic nerve leaves via the optic disc.

image of the object falls directly on to the fovea. This is why only the very centre of an area at which you are looking is seen clearly and why things at the edge of the field of vision tend to be hazy.

All the ganglion cell axons are gathered together in the optic nerve which leaves through the back of the retina. At the point where the optic nerve leaves the eyeball there are no rods or cones and so if light falls on this area it cannot be detected. This is known as the blind spot.

COLOUR VISION. Light can be regarded as consisting of waves. The wavelength of light, the distance from the peak of one wave to the peak of the next determines the colour which we see. The eye as a whole can detect light waves whose wave lengths range from about 400 to about 700 mu (1 mu is one thousand millionth of a metre). Visual purple can be broken down by light of any wavelength within this range and so the rods can see only one 'colour'. The cones are quite different. There are three distinct types, each of which is specialized to detect light of a much more limited range of wavelengths. Blue light has short wavelengths near the 400 mu end. Green light has medium length wavelengths in the 500–600 mu range Red light has relative long wavelengths in the 600–700 mu range.

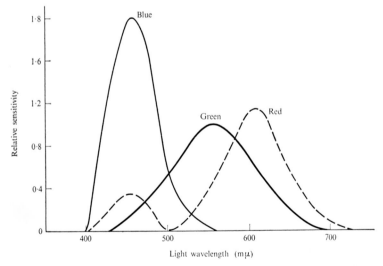

Fig.2.28. The three types of cone which are believed to be important in colour vision. Each is particularly sensitive to light of a limited wavelength.

The three types of cones are each specialized to detect light of a particular type. The pigment in the 'blue' cones is broken down by light in the blue wavelength range and so the blue cones will fire impulses when blue light falls upon them but not when red light reaches them. The 'red' cones have a pigment which is broken down by light of the red wavelength range but not by blue light. They will therefore fire impulses when red light falls on them. The 'green' cones have a pigment which is intermediate between the two.

If you have ever taken any interest in theatre lighting you wil know that you can produce light of any colour, including white by using three lamps, one red, one green and one blue. When all three lamps are shining on a spot with equal intensity, the whole range of visible wavelengths is represented and the result is white. All the other colours may be made by altering the intensities of the three lights. Colour vision works in a roughly similar way. If only red light falls on the retina, only the 'red' cones will fire impulses. Nothing will happen in the green and blue cones and the brain can therefore 'know' that the light falling on the eye must be red. Similarly, if pure green or pure blue light falls on the retina, only the relevant cones will be stimulated and the brain can know what colour the light must be. If white light, which contains all the wavelengths from 400 to 700 mu falls on the retina, all three cones will be firing equally. The brain will note that all the cones are firing, that the light must therefore contain all wavelengths and that it must therefore be white. Other colours are formed by different patterns of cone firing. A yellow sensation, for example, occurs when the green cones are firing rapidly and the red ones are firing moderately. This is because yellow light has a wavelength between green and red light but which is closer to green. An orange light on the other hand produces rapid firing of the red cones and moderate firing of the green cones. This is because orange light has a wavelength which is closer to red than to green. Thus by looking at the pattern of firing in the different types of cone the brain can know the colour of light which is falling on the retina.

DARK ADAPTATION. When you go from the light outside into a darkened room you are all familiar with the sensation of being quite unable to see anything because there is not enough light reaching your eyes. Gradually, as you become accustomed to the gloom, you can see more and more: your vision continues to improve for about 25 minutes after which no further improvement takes place.

No matter how long you stay in the dark you cannot see colours. although you may be able to see things quite clearly in shades of grey. This process is known as dark adaptation.

The sequence of events in dark adaptation depends on two facts. First, in ordinary daylight or in bright artificial light, the brightness of the light is sufficient to break down all the visual purple which is immediately available. Since if there is no intact visual purple to be broken down the rods cannot detect light, the rods are functionless in bright conditions. Secondly, the cone pigments are much less sensitive than visual purple. They are more resistant to being broken down and they cannot detect light whose intensity is below a critical level. So in the bright surroundings the rods are functionless because the bright light has broken down the visual purple and you rely entirely on cone vision. When you go into a dark room, the cones cannot work because the light intensity is too low, while the rods cannot work because they do not contain enough available visual purple. You are therefore temporarily blind. But as soon as the bright light is removed, visual purple begins to be manufactured again in the rods and as its concentration rises so the rods again become sensitive to light. The process continues for about 25 minutes when the maximum sensitivity is reached.

An interesting phenomenon which you may have noticed is that at night when you try to look directly at an object such as a star, it seems to disappear. When you look a little to one side, the object appears again. This occurs because when you look directly at something, the image falls on the fovea where there are only cones: since the cones are functionless in dim light at night you cannot see objects whose image falls on the fovea. But if you look to one side the image falls not on the fovea but on a part of the retina which contains rods and you can see the object again. When you are trying to see something at night it therefore pays not to look directly at it.

COLOUR BLINDNESS. Some people cannot distinguish between colours in the normal way. This is because instead of having three types of cone they have only one or two. This means that it is difficult or impossible for such individuals to distinguish between certain colours: the difficulties vary depending on the cones which are missing, but the commonest one is a difficulty in distinguishing between red and green.

The normal function of cones seems to depend on genes which are carried on the X chromosome. In females there are two X chromosomes but in males there is only one. In females it is possible for one X chromosome to be defective, but so long as the other X

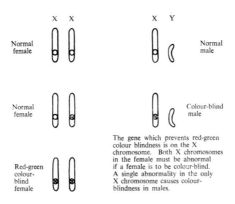

Fig.2.29. The inheritance of colour blindness.

chromosome is normal, colour vision will be normal. In females the common forms of colour blindness will occur only if both X chromosomes are defective. In males, however, with only one X chromosome, there is no such safety factor. If that single chromosome is defective, colour blindness will occur. This explains why the common form of red-green colour blindness is so much more common in males than in females.

EYE MOVEMENTS AND VISUAL FIELDS. Normally the two eyes move together so that the image of a particular object falls on the fovea of each eye simultaneously. In other words the two eyes look at the same thing and the two separate images are fused into one by processes which occur in the brain. If the two eyes do not look at the same point at the same time, the person is said to have strabismus or a squint. Double vision may occur, but is often absent because the brain totally ignores the information coming from the abnormal eye and takes notice only of the normal one.

Because of the nose and the margins of the eye sockets, the area seen by one eye is not exactly the same as that seen by the other eye. The area seen by one eye is known as the visual field of that eye. You can easily confirm that the two visual fields are slightly different by looking straight ahead and shutting each eye in turn. The assessment of visual fields is an important part of the examination of a patient because it may reveal damage to the eyes, to the optic nerves or to the brain.

In order to understand why the visual fields should be tested it is important to know the pathways which the nerves take from the eyes to the occipital cortex. These are shown in Fig.2.30. The first

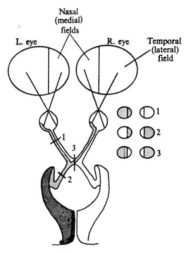

Fig.2.30. The visual pathways from the eye to the visual cortex and the effects on the visual fields of cuts at various points.

thing to note is that the light rays cross over in the focussing system, so that the image of objects on the right side of the body falls on the left side of the eye and vice versa. Secondly, the nerve fibres from the outer (lateral) half of each retina go to the same side of the brain, while those from the inner (medial) half of each retina cross over in the optic chiasma and go to the opposite side of the brain. In Fig.2.30 various cuts are shown and the explanation of the damage which each one causes is given below.

1. This cut severs the optic nerve on one side before the optic chiasma. Thus all the fibres coming from one eye will be destroyed and total blindness will occur on that side. The visual field of the other eye will be normal.

2. This cuts the optic pathway behind the chiasma. It therefore destroys the fibres carrying information from the outer side of the

retina on the same side as the cut and those from the inner side of the retina on the opposite side to the cut. Thus if the cut is on the right side, all the fibres coming from the right sides of both eyes will be destroyed. Since the right side of each eye sees objects on the left side of the body, in each eye the left side of the visual field will be missing. If the cut is on the left side, the right side of each field will be defective.

3. This cuts the optic chiasma. Such damage could occur naturally as a result of the growth of a tumour of the pituitary gland which lies just below the chiasma. The fibres from the inner side of each retina will be destroyed. In the left eye the right side of the retina will be affected and so the eye will be unable to see objects on the left side of the body. Similarly the right eye will be unable to see objects on the right side of the body. When both eyes are open each eye will tend to compensate for the other's defects.

REFLEXES

All actions in some way depend on sensory information received by the CNS. The information may have been stored in the brain as a result of past experience as when a pianist plays a piece of music from memory. On the other hand the information may have been received immediately before the motor act, as when someone playing tennis moves to where she sees the ball is going. In many cases we are aware of what is going on and we consciously direct the motor action. In other cases, although we may be aware of what is happening, the motor response occurs involuntarily without our conscious direction, as when a hand is pulled away from an unexpectedly hot plate. In still other situations we neither direct the motor response consciously nor are aware that it is happening, as when the body regulates arterial pressure in order to cope with a fall or a rise in pressure. The last two examples are both known as reflexes. We can say that a reflex occurs whenever a sensory stimulus leads to a motor (effector) response without the intervention of conscious, voluntary control. In order for a reflex to occur, five essential components must be present:

1. A sensory receptor for detecting that the stimulus has occurred.

2. A sensory nerve fibre for carrying the information to the CNS.

3. A control centre in the CNS which collects the sensory informa-

tion and decides on appropriate motor action: at its simplest this centre may consist of a single synapse.

4. A motor nerve which carries information from the CNS to the appropriate effector.

5. An effector organ (usually a muscle or a gland) which carries out the response.

Reflexes vary a great deal in their complexity. The simplest can occur even after damage to the spinal cord has cut it off from the rest of the CNS. Such simple reflexes are known as spinal reflexes and have naturally been studied most in experimental animals. Nevertheless, they can also be clearly seen in patients whose spinal cord has been damaged by accident or by disease. The most important spinal reflexes are:

1. *The stretch reflex or tendon jerk.* This is best illustrated by the familiar response to tapping the front of the knee. The leg is allowed to hang freely and a sharp tap is given to the tendon which stretches from the knee cap to the tibia. This gives a brief stretch to the quadriceps muscle on top of the thigh. The stretch stimulates sensory receptors known as muscle spindles, which consist of specialized muscle fibres with sensory nerves wrapped around them. The sensory fibres carry the impulses up to the spinal cord. In the

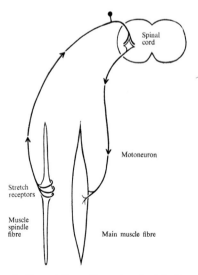

Fig.2.31. A muscle spindle and the pathway involved in the stretch reflex.

spinal cord the sensory fibres synapse with motoneurons which go back to the muscle which was stretched. The impulses going along these motoneurons cause the muscle to contract. Thus a brief stretch of any muscle is always normally followed by a brief contraction of the stretched muscle. One possible function of the stretch reflex will be discussed later under the heading of posture.

2. *The flexion reflex.* This is the response of a limb to a painful stimulus. Whenever any potentially damaging stimulus is applied to a limb, it is detected by pain receptors which send the information to the spinal cord. This leads at once to a coordinated movement of the limb in which the flexor muscles contract and the extensors relax, so pulling the limb away from the danger zone.

3. *The crossed extension reflex.* This is closely related to the flexion reflex. If you tread on something sharp and the flexion reflex pulls your leg up quickly, you will fall unless you are supported by your other leg. In fact you do not usually fall because the extensor muscles in the unstimulated leg contract so making the limb into a firm pillar on which you can stand. Thus a painful stimulus to one leg causes extension of the other leg and this is known as the crossed extension reflex.

4. *The response to stroking firmly the underside of the foot with a blunt point.* In a normal individual this causes curling up of the toes and in particular of the great toe. In someone whose motor pathway from the motor cortex to the spinal cord has been damaged, the great toe, instead of flexing downwards extends upwards. This is known as the Babinski response and is usually an indication of severe damage either to the spinal cord or to the motor tracts in the brain. The only exception to this rule is that the Babinski response is normal during the first 12–18 months of life before the spinal cord tracts have received their normal coats of myelin. The process of the myelination of the motor tracts continues for quite a long period after birth and is associated with the progressive development of the infant's motor behaviour.

5. *Micturition* (urination) in response to a full bladder. This occurs automatically in infants and in those whose spinal cord has been damaged above the lumbar region. In normal individuals the micturition reflex is, of course, brought under voluntary control.

6. *The defaecation reflex* is similar to the micturition reflex.

7. *Erection of the penis and ejaculation of sperm.* This can be

brought about after spinal cord section by stimulation of the glans of the penis. The person being stimulated cannot feel what is happening. However this reflex enables paraplegic patients (ones whose spinal cord has been cut across) to father children. The sperm can be collected and the wife fertilized by artificial insemination.

Many other reflexes operate to keep the body running smoothly but they require the participation of parts of the brain above the level of the spinal cord. Important examples of these more complex reflexes are:

1. The responses of the respiratory system to oxygen lack and carbon dioxide excess (chapter 6).

2. The responses of the cardiovascular system which help to maintain the constancy of the arterial pressure (chapter 5).

3. The control of the output of aldosterone and anti-diuretic hormone. These hormones modify the behaviour of the kidneys and help to keep the composition of the body fluids constant (chapter 7).

4. The reflexes involved in the maintenance of posture which are described later in this section.

Conditioned reflexes

All the reflexes so far described are inborn. They are possessed by every normal individual, develop automatically and do not have to be learned. Conditioned reflexes while also being involuntary motor acts in response to a sensory stimulus, are different in that they are acquired by experience. They were first clearly demonstrated by the Russian scientist Pavlov, using dogs. Dogs, like most animals, respond to the sight and smell of food by pouring out saliva. Pavlov devised a method of collecting this saliva and measuring its quantity. In a group of dogs, every time he provided food he simultaneously rang a bell. After he had given the food and rung the bell together a number of times, he then rang the bell without giving the food. The dogs still poured out saliva. They had come to associate the bell with the food and therefore salivated even when no food was provided: they thought that the bell was an indication that food would be coming. Daily life is full of examples of such conditioned reflexes. For example small children do not naturally refrain from running into the road when they hear the sound of a car engine. Only as they grow and gradually begin to associate cars with danger do they automatically jump off the road when they hear a car coming.

If you think a little you will find many other examples of acquired conditioned reflexes in your own life. They are reflexes in which a stimulus is not naturally associated with an involuntary response, but in which it becomes so as a result of experience.

SENSORY PATHWAYS IN THE CNS

We are not aware of much of the information which is continually being collected by our sense organs. Only a small proportion of the information reaches the level of consciousness. When sensory information is consciously appreciated it is said to be perceived. Perception is the being aware of a particular sensory event.

Sensory information is carried from the receptors to the brain and spinal cord by sensory nerves. In the CNS these nerves make contact with other nerve cells which carry the impulses up to the thalamus and to the cerebral cortex and to the cerebellum. There is some evidence that crude sensations are perceived at the thalamus, but that their precise localization and identification requires the participation of the cerebral cortex. For example, after destruction of the cerebral cortex which leaves the thalamus intact, it is possible to be aware that a painful stimulus has been applied to the body, but it is impossible to localize it precisely.

The routes via which the most important types of sensory information reach the brain are outlined in Fig.2.32.

1. Information about pain, temperature and pressure on the skin below the level of the neck. The sensory fibres enter the spinal cord and synapse immediately. The fibres of the spino-thalamic tract then cross to the other side of the spinal cord and carry the information up to the thalamus. These types of information do not appear to reach the cerebral cortex.

2. Information from below the neck about light touch to the skin, vibration and the position of the joints. The fibres from receptors enter the spinal cord and without synapsing travel up in the posterior columns of the cord to the posterior column nuclei at the junction of brain and cord. There they synapse and another set of fibres carries the impulses up to the thalamus of the opposite side. A third set of nerve cells then transmits the information to the sensory cortex.

3. Information of all types from the skin of the head enters the brain via the trigeminal nerve, is carried to the thalamus of the

opposite side. Light touch and vibration information is then carried up to the sensory cortex.

4. Information about sound enters the brain via the auditory nerve. Some is sent to the cerebral cortex on the same side and some to the opposite side. This means that each half of the brain receives information from both ears.

5. Information from the eyes was dealt with in an earlier section.

SENSORY AREAS OF THE CEREBRAL CORTEX

While vague sensations of light, sound, pain, touch and so on may probably be appreciated at the thalamic level, precise identification and localization of stimuli requires the participation of the cerebral cortex. Three main areas are involved. Dividing the cortex into

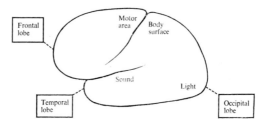

Fig.2.32. The sensory areas of the cerebral cortex.

anterior and posterior parts is a deep central fissure (sulcus). Immediately behind this is the area devoted to analysing information from the body surface and the joints. The body surface is not evenly and proportionally represented. For instance, the areas of the cortex devoted to the hands and to the lips are out of all proportion to the skin areas involved and are enormous compared to the cortical areas devoted to the trunk and to the legs. This is presumably because the hands and lips are exposed to a much greater variety of stimulation than the trunk and legs. The whole area of cortex which deals with the skin surface is sometimes known as the somatic sensory cortex. If it is destroyed on one side, sensation on the opposite side of the body is lost.

The part of the cortex which deals with vision, the visual cortex, is right at the back of the brain in the occipital region. The left occipital cortex receives information from the left side of each retina. The left side of each retina receives light from the right hand side of the body. Therefore if the left side of the occipital cortex is destroyed, a person looking straight ahead will be unable to see objects on his right.

The auditory cortex lies below the somatic sensory cortex in the temporal lobe of the brain. Each part of the auditory cortex receives information about sound from both ears and so damage to one side causes little if any hearing loss.

THE MOTOR CORTEX

The voluntary control of muscular activity depends to a large extent on the motor cortex which lies in front of the central sulcus. It is arranged in much the same way as the sensory cortex. Large areas are devoted to the hands and face which carry out a wide

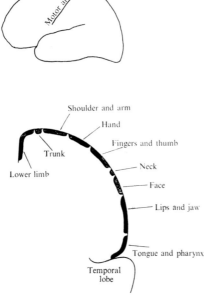

Fig.2.33. The position of the motor cortex and a coronal section through it showing the relative sizes of the areas which deal with muscles in different parts of the body.

range of delicate movements, while much smaller areas are devoted to the trunk and legs which carry out a much smaller range of relatively crude and stereotyped movements. Instructions about voluntary movements are sent down from the motor cortex by two systems of fibres, the pyramidal and the extra-pyramidal tracts. In the pyramidal tract, single continuous fibres go right from the motor cortex down to the motoneurons of the spinal cord. In the extra-pyramidal tract the information is carried by a chain of shorter neurons. Both tracts cross in the brain to the opposite side and so each half of the motor cortex deals with the opposite side of the body. Damage to the motor cortex therefore causes paralysis on the opposite side of the body.

OTHER ASPECTS OF CEREBRAL CORTICAL FUNCTION

The brain has many other functions apart from the ones which have so far been discussed. Some such as memory we are very far indeed from understanding and there is little point in dealing with them here. Other functions which we are just beginning to understand are sleep and speech and these will be discussed in this section.

Sleep

The electrical activity of the tens of millions of nerve cells of which the cerebral cortex is composed can be recorded through the skull. Sensitive electrodes placed at many points on the surface of the scalp can pick up this activity and feed it into a machine known as

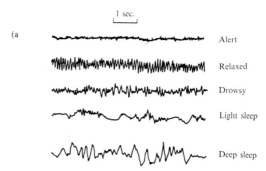

Fig.2.34a. Some typical EEGs showing the transition from the alert state to deep sleep.

(b)

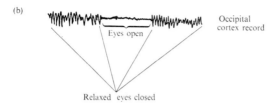

Occipital
cortex record

Eyes open

Relaxed eyes closed

Fig.2.34*b*. Opening the eyes abolishes the alpha rhythm seen in most normal adults when resting quietly with the eyes closed.

an electroencephalograph (EEG) or electrocorticograph. This amplifies the electrical signals and records them on moving paper.

When a person is awake and alert, the oscillations of electrical activity are very fast and irregular. When a person becomes drowsy and closes his eyes, the waves become slower and more coordinated giving the so-called alpha rhythm. On going to sleep the further changes shown in Fig.2.34 can be seen: large slow waves alternate with bursts of high frequency activity known as sleep spindles. The basic rhythm seen in a relaxed individual varies with age. In infancy slow delta rhythms of less than 4/second dominate. During childhood the theta rhythms (4–8/sec) predominate, gradually giving way to the mature alpha pattern (8–14/sec) after puberty. Apart from its use in experimental situations as an indicator of sleep, the EEG is of importance in four main situations:

1. In certain psychiatric behavioural disorders, the theta rhythms persist into adult life reflecting the immaturity of the personality of the patient.

2. In epilepsy, abnormal electrical discharges may be seen and the site of their origin identified.

3. Cerebral tumours, abscesses or other abnormalities within the skull may produce an abnormal EEG pattern.

4. The EEG may be used to try to decide whether a person's cortex is dead or alive. This may be important after injury or drug overdose when the heart may be beating normally but the brain (and therefore the person) may be dead.

The state of sleep seems to be controlled by a system of nerve cells in the core of the mid brain and hind brain known as the reticular formation or the reticular activating system. The reticular formation has connections with the whole cerebral cortex and its activity determines whether the person will be awake and conscious

3

or asleep and unconscious. Experiments with animals have shown that destruction of the reticular formation produces a permanent state of sleep while stimulation of it by means of electrodes implanted into it produces a permanently awake state. In humans, haemorrhage into the mid brain (pontine haemorrhage) damages the reticular formation and causes a state of deep unconsciousness from which the patient cannot be roused. Many sleeping pills, and in particular the barbiturates, seem to act by suppressing the activity of the reticular formation.

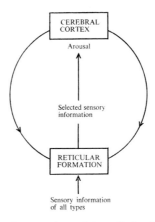

Fig.2.35. The function and connections of the reticular formation.

The reticular formation appears to work by collecting information from two major sources and using that information to regulate the activity of the cortex. The sources are:

1. The situation in the environment as determined by the activity of peripheral sensory organs. Everyone acknowledges the importance of this by trying to reduce sensory activity as much as possible before going to sleep. We switch off the radio and the light and try to ensure that the bed is neither too cold nor too hot. This cuts down the sensory information pouring into the reticular formation and reduces its activity.

2. The state of cortical activity. Again everyone is aware of the importance of this. Impending important events such as examinations, an exciting date or marriage keep us thinking even if the environ-

mental situation is ideal for sleep. The cortex remains active and the reticular formation will not allow us to go to sleep.

The reticular formation is more than a simple collector of information. It also assesses the significance of the information received. For example, if you live by a railway line you soon cease to be woken up by the trains running at night. Your reticular formation receives the information about the train from your ears in the usual way. However it soon learns that this information is of no importance and so does not bother to rouse the cortex and wake you up. Yet if your bedroom door creaks while a train is thundering past you are awake in an instant. The reticular formation has decided that the small sound of the creaking door may be very important and has aroused the cortex to activity. The reticular information therefore receives all the information coming from sensory organs, but it acts to arouse the cortex only if the information seems important.

Speech

The ability to speak involves a remarkably complex series of processes. First, it is important to understand what words are and what they mean. Second, the words which are appropriate to a particular situation must be selected. Third, instructions must be sent to the muscles of the chest, the larynx and the mouth in order that they may produce the required sounds. It is not surprising that we are only just beginning to understand how the brain deals with speech.

The use of words is clearly closely involved with the hearing of sound and with the seeing of the printed page. It also involves the control of muscles of the chest, larynx, throat and mouth. It is therefore not surprising that the area of the cerebral cortex which deals with speech lies between the three areas which deal with sight, with hearing and with muscular activity. It has been found that in most individuals it is the dominant hemisphere which is most important in speech. Thus in right handed individuals in whom the left hemisphere is dominant speech depends primarily on the function of the left hemisphere. In left handed individuals speech depends on the right hemisphere. There is some evidence that many people who stammer are naturally left handed but in childhood were forced to become right handed by parents or teachers who mistakenly thought that right handedness was somehow better. This attempt to change the dominant hemisphere by outside action obviously must have serious consequences for the organization of the brain, leading to problems in speaking.

There are three relatively simple disorders which lead to problems in word use. Blindness makes it impossible to read with the eyes although it may be possible so to develop the sense of touch that the Braille symbols can be interpreted as letters. Deafness makes it impossible to hear sounds and in the development of speech is a much more important defect than blindness. Deaf children cannot hear speech and cannot naturally learn to speak. Unless they receive special education they remain dumb. Dysarthria is an inability to formulate sounds properly because of some damage to the motor cortex or motor pathways which interfere with the normal control of muscular activity. In none of these situations is there any real difficulty in the understanding and choosing of words.

Aphasia is a much more complex problem: it is a condition which results from damage to the speech area in the dominant cerebral hemisphere, often as a result of a cerebrovascular accident or stroke. The patient has difficulty in understanding words, in arranging them in their correct order and in selecting the ones which he wants to use. As can be imagined this is a very distressing condition since it makes it extremely difficult for anyone to communicate with the patient.

HYPOTHALAMUS

The hypothalamus, as its name implies, lies beneath the thalamus at the base of the fore brain. It is a region which is currently being much investigated because it seems to be the site involved in much of emotional and sexual behaviour. In animals, stimulation of the hypothalamus by electric currents can cause uncontrollable rage or perfect calm, fear or aggression, eagerness to mate or lack of interest in sex. As yet we know very little about the significance of these things in humans. Certainly some tumours of the hypothalamus can result in very strange human behaviour, but such tumours are rare and difficult to study.

The hypothalamus is also important because it controls the behaviour of the pituitary gland, the so-called 'master gland' in the body. The pituitary receives blood via a special system of vessels from the hypothalamus. The hypothalamus secretes into this blood releasing factors which alter the secretion rates of the anterior pituitary hormones. In this way the hypothalamus controls growth, the thyroid, the adrenal and the gonads.

POSTURE AND MOVEMENT. THE CEREBELLUM

One of the most important functions of the nervous system is the control of muscular activity. But it is a mistake to think that this control depends only on the motor side of the system. The sensory side is just as important. This is clearly illustrated by considering the difference between playing tennis with your eyes shut and your eyes open. When the motor system is deprived of sensory information it becomes almost useless. Only if it receives a continuous supply of reliable sensory information can the motor system work safely and effectively.

A major part of the work of the motor system concerns the maintenance of posture, particularly when you are standing up. The important sensory receptors which provide the brain with information about posture are as follows:

1. The eyes. These provide a constant stream of information about the position of the body, of the head, of the limbs and about objects in the environment.

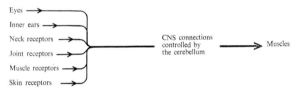

Fig.2.36. Outline of the systems involved in the control of posture.

2. The labyrinths in the inner ear. These provide information about the position and the movements of the head.

3. Receptors in the joints of the neck. These supply information about the position of the head in relation to that of the body.

4. Receptors in other joints. These provide information about the position of the limbs. Conscious knowledge of limb position depends on these joint receptors and not on receptors in muscles.

5. Receptors in the muscles known as muscle spindles and Golgi tendon organs. These provide the CNS with information about muscle stretch and contraction, but we are not consciously aware of it.

6. Skin receptors which provide information as to which part of the skin is taking the weight of the body.

All this information is made available to the motor areas of the brain and is continually put to use as the CNS directs muscular activity. Of all the receptors, the most important are the eyes. However, damage to any one set of receptors may lead to disturbances in posture, especially when the eyes cannot be used properly as in blind people or in the dark.

The cerebellum

One of the most formidable problems faced by the nervous system is that of precisely controlling the strength of muscular contraction in the face of the very variable amounts of force which must be used. For example, how does the body solve the problem of lifting a suitcase of unknown weight, of pushing open a swing door whose springs offer unknown resistance, or of perpetually operating against gravity which puts a continual limitation on movement? We understand very little about the details, but the answers seem to lie in the functioning of the cerebellum which lies attached to the hind brain just above the spinal cord. The cerebellum receives a steady supply of all the information which could conceivably be of importance in muscle movement. Using this information it modifies the instructions sent out by the motor cortex, so that the power of muscular activity is continually adjusted to cope with varying opposing forces.

The cerebellum is different from most other parts of the brain in that each side of it receives information from and controls the same side of the body, not the opposite side as in the case of the cortex. The left hand side of the motor cortex controls the right hand side of the body, but the left hand side of the cerebellum controls the left hand side of the body. Damage to the left side of the cerebellum leads to weakness on the left side of the body. As a result, when a person with such damage walks, he veers to the left because the right leg takes normal steps while the left leg takes small ones. In contrast the patient tends to look to his right: this is because the muscles on the right side of the neck are working normally while those on the left are weak and so the head is pulled to the right. The reverse situations will occur if the right side of the cerebellum is damaged.

Normally movements are smooth because the cerebellum continually adjusts the strength of muscle contraction to deal with the resistance which the muscles meet. These adjustments are carried out entirely subconsciously and depend on information from the muscles and joints and many other receptors. If the cerebellum is damaged, the smooth adjustments no longer take place and movements become jerky as the person has to adjust the strength of muscle contraction consciously. In a person with cerebellar damage, the muscles show no tremor (shaking) at rest, but as soon as movement begins a jerkiness or tremor appears. Because this occurs only on movement it is sometimes known as 'Intention tremor'. A good test which usually clearly shows up intention tremor is to ask the patient to touch the tip of his nose with his forefinger. As you can demonstrate on yourself a normal person can do this quickly and smoothly either with eyes shut or with eyes open. Someone with cerebellar damage may just succeed when his eyes are open, but the movement will be slow and jerky and will become jerkier and jerkier as the nose is approached and precise adjustments are required. With eyes shut a person with cerebellar damage usually completely fails to touch his nose: this is because in the absence of the cerebellum he relies entirely on his eyes to tell him about the progress of a movement.

Like all other muscles, those of the larynx, mouth and face are also controlled by the cerebellum. In people with cerebellar damage the movements of these muscles cannot be regulated precisely and speech becomes slurred (dysarthria).

One part of the cerebellum, known as the flocculonodular lobe, is particularly concerned with the maintenance of the upright posture. If it is damaged the person finds it impossible to stand upright, even though while he is sitting the muscle movements of arms and head are normal. There is a tumour of small children known as a medulloblastoma which characteristically starts in the flocculonodular lobe. The first indication of its presence is usually difficulty in standing upright, even though muscle movements when lying in bed are more or less normal.

Muscle spindles and posture

Muscle spindles are also important in the maintenance of normal posture. As we saw earlier when discussing the 'knee jerk' when a muscle is stretched, the muscle spindles in that muscle discharge impulses which travel to the spinal cord. There they synapse with the motoneurons going back to the same muscle that is stretched. A burst of impulses is therefore fired along these motoneurons and the muscle contracts. This reflex is important in helping you to stand upright. If when standing you sway forwards, the muscles in the back and on the back of the legs are slightly stretched. This activates the muscle spindles and as a result a reflex occurs which makes those muscles contract and brings you back to the upright position. If you sway forwards or to one side, similar events occur which bring you upright again. The muscle spindles and the reflex they initiate are therefore important in the maintenance of posture.

Basal ganglia

These are a group of nerve centres in the fore brain near the thalamus. Their function is poorly understood but it is certain that like the cerebellum, they have an important role to play in the maintenance of posture and the regulation of movement. They are important in medicine because it seems that the basal ganglia are at fault in the very common condition known as Parkinson's disease. This disease is characterized by the following three major features:

1. Muscle stiffness. The limbs are stiff and difficult to move and in the face this appears as a 'woodenness' of expression.

2. Difficulty in maintaining the upright position with a tendency to fall frequently.

3. Tremor, which in contrast to that of cerebellar disease is present at rest even when the patient is not attempting to carry out any movement.

The condition may sometimes be considerably improved by surgical destruction of some of the basal ganglia which appear to be malfunctioning. It has been suggested that it may be due to a deficiency of a chemical in the brain known as L-DOPA and treatment with this drug has recently given encouraging results.

DAMAGE TO THE NERVOUS SYSTEM

There are innumerable forms of damage to the nervous system but here I shall discuss only three common ones where a knowledge of physiology is particularly helpful in understanding what happens.

Peripheral nerve damage

When a peripheral nerve is cut, stimuli which fall on the area of skin which that nerve supplies can no longer be felt. The muscles supplied by that nerve are paralysed and can no longer contract in either voluntary or reflex movements. They become totally flabby (flaccid). The muscle may undergo spontaneous irregular contractions as a result of impulses being fired off in the irritated cut end of the nerve, but unless regeneration of the nerve occurs the muscle will eventually atrophy and all the contractile tissue will be replaced by fat.

Loss of nerve supply to the skin causes the skin to become shiny and to lose elasticity: it is taut and easily damaged. The mechanism of this skin change is unknown but it may be partly caused by lack of secretion of the glands in the skin.

If the two ends of a cut nerve can be sewn together some recovery may occur. The central end of the nerve remains alive because it is still connected to the cell bodies in or near the spinal cord. The peripheral part dies but the tubes which contained the nerve axons remain. If regeneration takes place, new axons growing from the end may travel down the empty tubes and eventually reach the nerve endings and re-establish function. However, regeneration is a slow process and complete recovery is extremely unlikely. This is obvious from the fact that a nerve the thickness of the pin may contain 100,000 fibres: for effective function each fibre must travel from the spinal cord to a particular part of the skin, to a particular muscle or to a particular gland without interruption. It is obvious that if the two ends of a cut nerve are stitched together only a tiny proportion of the fibres will succeed in making the right connections.

Regeneration of nerves is often such a prolonged process that by the time even a few fibres reach a muscle, the muscle has atrophied. In order to prevent this, physiotherapists may stimulate a muscle by giving direct electric shocks to it. This does not completely prevent atrophy but the regular contractions slow down the process considerably.

Spinal cord section

Complete transection of the spinal cord produces total paralysis of voluntary movement and total absence of conscious sensation at points innervated from below the level of the injury. No nerve regeneration at all occurs in the CNS and if the cord has truly been severed the damage is permanent. Such a condition where the lower part of the body is paralysed while the upper part is normal is known as paraplegia.

Immediately after damage to the spinal cord not only can the muscles not be moved voluntarily, they do not move in response to reflexes and are completely paralysed and flaccid. This situation of total unresponsiveness of muscles is known as spinal shock. It lasts only a few minutes in the frog, an hour or so in cats and dogs and two to six weeks in man. During this period no reflexes can be demonstrated. The bladder fills but does not empty and must be drained by means of a catheter. Similarly faeces must be removed manually from the rectum because defaecation does not take place. Eventually however the spinal shock passes off and in most cases the reflexes listed below return.

1. Babinski response. This is a sign of damage to the pyramidal tract and has already been discussed.

2. Flexion reflex. This is often very troublesome as it may become hypersensitive. Normally it is set off only by painful stimuli, but in paraplegics it may be initiated by very minor things such as bread-crumbs in the bed or ingrowing toe nails. Although the patient cannot feel pain, violent flexion reflexes may throw him around the bed.

3. Micturition. When the bladder fills to a certain critical level it empties automatically as in an infant. The patient may be able to achieve some control over micturition as in some paraplegics the reflex may be initiated by scratching or pressing on the anterior abdominal wall, thus enabling the patient to micturate at a convenient time.

4. Defaecation. This too becomes automatic. A few patients may be able to initiate it by pressing hard on the abdomen to increase the intra-abdominal pressure.

5. Ejaculation of sperm. Mechanical stimulation of the penis may produce erection and ejaculation even though the patient can feel nothing. If the sperm is collected it can then be used for artificial insemination of the wife so that a paraplegic patient may have children.

6. Stretch reflex (tendon jerk). In the later stages of recovery this too may become over-excitable. As a result the limbs become very stiff and resistant to bending and the tendon jerks become greatly exaggerated. This condition is known as spasticity.

Cerebrovascular accident (CVA) or stroke

A stroke is caused by damage to the brain resulting from blockage of an artery, by a clot, or from the rupture of an artery with resulting haemorrhage. The damaged area is most commonly in the region of the tracts coming down from the motor cortex and going up to the sensory cortex. As a result, the patient loses voluntary movement and conscious sensation on the opposite side of the body. This situation, where say the right half of the body is damaged while the left half is normal, is known as hemiplegia in contrast to the paraplegia which results from spinal section. The main features of hemiplegia apart from loss of voluntary movement and conscious sensation, are spasticity and a Babinski response on the affected side. Speech is very commonly affected. If the non-dominant cerebral hemisphere is affected, the defect is likely to be dysarthria because the motor control of the muscles is abnormal but the understanding and use of words is normal. If the dominant hemisphere is affected, however, the patient may have trouble in understanding and selecting words in addition to the motor defect: this more serious situation is known as aphasia.

If the stroke occurs lower down in the brain in the region of the pons, the normal functioning of the reticular formation may be abolished. As a result the patient may lapse into a deep and permanent state of unconsciousness.

PAIN

The sensation of pain depends on the activation of fine nerve endings which can be found throughout the body. These fire off impulses whenever tissue damage has occurred or is about to occur. The usual stimuli which cause pain are extremes of heat and cold and mechanical stimulation and certain types of chemical damage such as erosion by acid. The impulses are carried to the spinal cord by sensory nerves which synapse with the fibres of the spinothalamic tract. The tract immediately crosses to the opposite side of the spinal cord and travels up to the thalamus.

All sensations have what may be called factual and emotional components. A touch on your hand activates the same receptors no matter who is doing the touching: that is the factual component. But your reaction to the touch depends very much on who is doing the touching: that is the emotional component and it depends on your assessment of the significance for your life of a factual event.

Pain has a very strong emotional component. Not only are we aware of the fact of a painful stimulus but we are also aware that it may mean discomfort, illness or even death. In some cases the emotional component of pain may be over-ruled by even stronger emotional circumstances and there are many examples of this in war and in sport. A soldier in battle or a footballer in an important match may be quite unaware of quite severe injuries: the man realizes that they have happened only when all the excitement is over. This demonstrates that the intensity of the pain sensation depends a great deal on the circumstances. Severe pain in the leg due to cramp is annoying but not emotionally disturbing: pain of a similar intensity in the chest may throw the patient into an acute anxiety state because he knows that it may mean a heart attack and death.

It therefore follows that in relieving pain two quite different things must be done:

1. The patient must be reassured that he is in good hands and that the cause of the pain is being dealt with calmly, quickly and effectively. This reassurance may be aided by giving sedative drugs which dull the patient's awareness of the significance of the pain.

2. Specific pain-relieving drugs may be given. These fall into four main categories:

   a. Those which are temperature-lowering (antipyretic) as well as pain-relieving (analgesic). Aspirin (acetyl salicylic acid) is the most used member of this group although there are many others. They relieve pain partly by acting directly on pain receptors and partly by acting on the brain.

   b. Those which are sleep-inducing (narcotic) as well as analgesic. Morphine and heroin come into this group. They are effective because they both allay fear and also dull the factual component of the pain, probably by acting on the parts of the brain which deal with pain.

   c. Local anaesthetics. These act directly on the peripheral nerves which carry information about pain. They block nerve conduction and are mainly used in dentistry and for the stitching of minor wounds.

   d. Anaesthetics which relieve pain by producing total unconsciousness. These are used for surgical operations.

Surgical relief of pain

Sometimes, particularly in patients with intractable cancer, pain may be so severe and persistent that drugs become ineffective. In these patients surgical procedures on the nervous system may be considered. There are three main types of operation:

1. Destruction of the spino-thalamic tract by cutting the antero-lateral part of the spinal cord where the tract runs. This operation is known as antero-lateral cordotomy.

2. Destruction of the part of the thalamus associated with pain. This is usually done by passing long needle electrodes into the thalamus and then passing strong electric currents through them in order to destroy brain tissue in the vicinity of the tip.

3. Pre-frontal leucotomy. This severs the connections between the frontal part of the cerebral cortex and the rest of the CNS. The operation does not interfere with the factual part of pain sensation, but it does alter its emotional component. The patient still feels the pain but is no longer unduly worried by it. The operation is sometimes done in other conditions, notably severe depression but it is now tending to fall out of use.

Referred and projected pain

Two other types of pain are important for the nurse and doctor. They are referred pain and projected pain. With referred pain, pain which really originates in some deep structure is felt somewhere on the skin surface: it is said to be 'referred' to the skin. There are many examples of this, but some important ones are:

1. Pain arising in the heart may be felt in the neck, the jaw, the shoulders (particularly the left) and down the inside of the left arm.

2. Pain arising from injury to or inflammation of the diaphragm (the sheet of muscle dividing chest from abdomen) may be referred to the tip of the shoulder.

3. In the early stages of appendicitis, pain arising from the inflamed appendix may be referred to the umbilicus.

4. Pain arising from the hip joint may be referred to the knee.

Referred pain seems to occur because there are more pain fibres in peripheral nerves than there are in the spino-thalamic tract. Thus several peripheral nerves, some from deep structures and some from the skin, must share the same spino-thalamic fibre. During life, skin

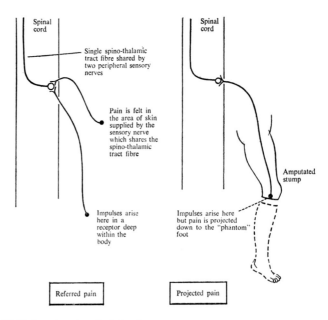

Fig.2.37. Referred and projected pain.

pain receptors are activated much more frequently than deep ones, so that the thalamus comes to associate pain in a particular spino-thalamic fibre with injury to the skin. When pain does arise in a deep structure it may be the first time in fifty or sixty years that the deep pain receptors have been activated: for example pain receptors in the heart are not activated until angina or a coronary thrombosis occurs. As a result the thalamus tends to refer the pain to the skin.

Projected pain is the pain which arises whenever the pain pathway is cut or damaged somewhere on its route from the pain receptor to the thalamus. A good example is that after amputation of a leg, the patient may complain that his foot is hurting (phantom limb pain). This is a very real sensation: the pain is genuinely felt and the patient must not be dismissed as a fraud. The pain occurs because the cut ends of nerves in the limb stump continue to fire impulses for some time. The brain 'knows' that impulses in those fibres normally come from pain receptors in the foot and so the pain is 'projected' to the foot and actually felt there. Another good example of projected pain is sciatica, when pressure on the sciatic nerve as it leaves the vertebral column at the bottom of the back fires off impulses in pain fibres in the nerve. The brain 'knows' that impulses in those fibres normally come from receptors in the back of the leg and so the pain is projected down the back of the leg.

AUTONOMIC NERVOUS SYSTEM
AND THE ADRENAL MEDULLA

All the motor nerves going to skeletal muscles are capable of being brought under voluntary control. A single nerve fibre goes right from the spinal cord to the muscle it supplies. In contrast, with a few exceptions, the motor nerves which control the behaviour of smooth muscle and of glands are not usually under voluntary control. These latter nerves make up the autonomic nervous system. They also differ from skeletal muscle nerves (sometimes called somatic nerves) in that there are usually at least two nerve fibres for carrying the impulses between the spinal cord and the muscle or gland.

The autonomic nervous system itself is divided into two main divisions, sympathetic and parasympathetic.

1. *Parasympathetic.* This arises from the brain and from the sacral region of the spinal cord. The main parasympathetic nerve arising in the brain is the vagus. The most important actions of the parasympathetic system are on the eye, the heart rate, the gut, the bladder and the reproductive organs. The nerve fibre which leaves the CNS is always very long and carries the parasympathetic impulses right to the organ where they will act. In the organ there is a synapse and the impulses are transmitted to a second short fibre which then goes to a muscle or to a gland cell. The chemical transmitter released by both first and second fibres is acetyl choline.

2. *Sympathetic.* This arises from the thoracic and lumbar regions of the spinal cord. The first nerve fibre is short and travels to one of the sympathetic ganglia (a ganglion is a collection of synapses) which lie in two chains, one on either side of the vertebral column. There are some additional ganglia in the mid-line, the most important of which is the coeliac plexus which lies in front of the aorta where the coeliac artery leaves the aorta. The chemical transmitter in the ganglia which carries the impulses from the first to the second neurons in the pathway, is again acetyl choline. The sympathetic fibres which leave the ganglia (post-ganglionic fibres) then go to smooth muscle and gland cells where they almost all act by releasing

noradrenaline. The main exceptions to this rule are the sympathetic fibres to the sweat glands which release acetyl choline.

The adrenal medulla

An endocrine gland which is very closely associated with the sympathetic system is the adrenal medulla, the inner part of the adrenal gland. The outer part, the adrenal cortex, has quite different functions as it is very much part of the endocrine system, and produces three different groups of steroid hormones, the mineralo-corticoids, glucocorticoids and the androgens. The adrenal medulla is supplied by pre-ganglionic sympathetic fibres which come straight from the spinal cord without synapsing. They release acetyl choline which stimulates the adrenal medulla to secrete its two hormones, adrenaline and noradrenaline.

Actions of the autonomic system

The main actions of the autonomic nervous system and the adrenal medulla are summarized in Table 2.1. One problem is that adrenaline seems to have two quite different groups of actions on smooth muscle. It makes many smooth muscle fibres, such as those in skin blood vessels, contract while it makes others, such as those in the bronchi and in muscle blood vessels, relax. Noradrenaline in contrast seems to be purely excitatory, making all types of smooth muscle contract. A synthetic substance, isoprenaline (isoproterenol) makes all smooth muscle fibres relax.

It is now apparent that muscle fibres contain two different types of keys or receptors on to which adrenaline, noradrenaline, iso-prenaline and related substances can become attached. These receptors have been called alpha (α) and beta (β). In general, α receptors cause muscle contraction while β receptors cause muscle relaxation. The structure of the noradrenaline molecule is such that it can occupy only α receptors and can only cause excitation. The isoprenaline molecule can occupy only β receptors and can only cause relaxation. Adrenaline, however, can occupy both α and β receptors and the overall effect which it has depends on whether there are more α receptors or more β receptors on that muscle. In lung smooth muscle, the β receptors predominate and so adrenaline causes relaxation. In skin arterioles, α receptors predominate and so adrenaline causes contraction.

Table 2.1. The actions of the autonomic nervous system and circulating adrenaline. Circulating adrenaline can activate both alpha and beta receptors but noradrenaline released from sympathetic nerves activates only alpha receptors. ACh indicates acetyl choline.

Structure	Receptor type	Sympathetic	Parasympathetic
Heart S-A node	Beta	Increases heart rate	—
	ACh	—	Slows the heart
Heart muscle	Beta	Increases contractility	—
Muscle arterioles	Alpha and beta	Constriction (noradrenaline) Dilatation (adrenaline)	
Skin, gut and kidney arterioles	Alpha	Constriction	
Bronchial muscle	Beta	Relaxation	—
	ACh	—	Contraction
Bronchial glands	ACh	—	Secretion
Main gut muscle	Beta	Relaxation	—
	ACh	—	Contraction
Salivary glands	Alpha	Mucus secretion	—
	ACh	—	Watery secretion
Gastric glands	ACh	—	Secretion
Pancreas	ACh	—	Secretion
Sweat glands	ACh	Secretion	—
Bladder wall	Beta	Relaxation	—
	ACh	—	Contraction
Sphincter of bladder	Alpha	Contraction	—
	ACh	—	Relaxation
Male sex organs	?	Ejaculation	Erection

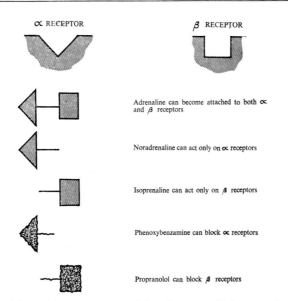

Fig.2.38. Alpha and beta receptors and the substances which act on them.

There is one important exception to the rule that β receptors are inhibitory and α receptors excitatory. This is that the β receptors in the heart which help to control heart rate are excitatory. Adrenaline and isoprenaline both therefore increase the rate of beating of the heart.

3

The body fluids

In a lean adult male, about 60 per cent of the body weight consists of water. Fatty tissue contains very little water and so as the amount of fat in the body rises, so the proportion of body weight made up of water falls. Females are almost always rather fatter than males and so in a normal female 50–55 per cent of the body weight consists of water. In an extremely obese person irrespective of sex, the water content may fall to 40 per cent of the body weight.

The total body water is divided into two major compartments, the water within cells (intra-cellular water) and that outside cells (extra-cellular water). About 55 per cent of the water is intra-cellular and about 45 per cent is extra-cellular. The extra-cellular water is further split up as follows:

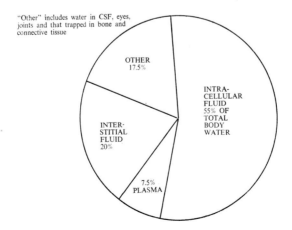

"Other" includes water in CSF, eyes, joints and that trapped in bone and connective tissue

OTHER 17.5%

INTRA-CELLULAR FLUID 55% OF TOTAL BODY WATER

INTER-STITIAL FLUID 20%

7.5% PLASMA

Fig.3.1. The main body fluid compartments.

1. Inside the blood vessels in the plasma: 7–8 per cent.

2. Interstitial fluid and lymph: 20 per cent.

3. Other compartments: 7–8 per cent. This includes the cerebrospinal fluid, the fluid in the eyes, water bound to bone, water bound to connective tissue and fluid in the joints.

CAPILLARY FUNCTION

In medicine it is particularly important to understand the balance between the plasma, the interstitial fluid (fluid between the cells and outside the blood vessels) and the lymph. Most of the blood vessels are impermeable to the passage of water and dissolved solids across their walls. It is only the tiniest blood vessels, the capillaries with walls a single cell thick, which allow fluid and dissolved material to pass from plasma to interstitial fluid and vice versa.

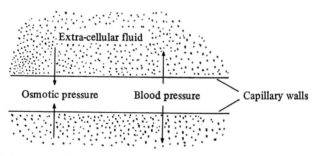

Fig.3.2. In a normal capillary there is an approximately even balance between the blood pressure and osmotic pressure.

Since the blood volume normally remains approximately constant, it is clear that the amount of fluid lost from the plasma into the interstitial fluid and the amount entering the plasma from the interstitial fluid must be evenly balanced. How is this balance maintained? Three major factors must be considered (a discussion of the basic physico-chemical concepts involved can be found in Essential Physics, Chemistry and Biology):

1. *The permeability of the capillary wall.* This is normally freely permeable to water, to ions such as those of sodium, chloride and

bicarbonate, and to small organic molecules such as those of glucose, amino acids and free fatty acids. In contrast, it will not permit the plasma proteins to pass through. In effect, all the constituents of blood apart from the cells and the protein can freely pass out of capillaries into the interstitial fluid.

2. *Protein osmotic pressure.* Because the protein cannot cross the capillary wall and because there is virtually no protein in the interstitial fluid, the plasma proteins exert an osmotic pressure which tends to draw water from the interstitial fluid into the blood.

3. *Blood pressure.* The pressure of the blood in the capillaries is much higher than that of the interstitial fluid. This pressure therefore tends to force fluid from the blood out into the interstitial fluid.

Under normal circumstances, there is an approximate balance between the blood pressure pushing fluid out of the capillaries and the plasma protein osmotic pressure drawing fluid back in. The blood pressure tends to be higher than the osmotic pressure at the arterial end of a capillary and so fluid there tends to move out. At the venous end of the capillary the blood pressure has fallen and the osmotic pressure, which has remained unchanged, is usually higher than the blood pressure. This results in fluid being drawn back into the blood.

THE LYMPH

Usually the blood pressure pushes out of the capillaries very slightly more fluid than the osmotic pressure of the proteins draws back in. This means that fluid tends slowly to move out of the blood into the interstitial fluid. If a disaster is not to occur, this fluid must somehow be returned to the blood and this is where the lymphatic system comes in.

The lymphatic system is a blind ended system of tubes ramifying to all parts of the body. Its finest branches, the lymphatic capillaries are like the blood capillaries in consisting of a single layer of cells. Unlike the blood capillaries they have very permeable walls and any protein which is in the interstitial fluid can freely enter the lymph. Particles of dirt, red and white blood cells, bacteria and cancer cells can also gain entry to the lymphatic capillaries. The lymphatic capillaries collect not only fluid but all sorts of foreign or waste material which gains entry to the interstitial fluid. In a way the lymphatic vessels therefore act as a drainage system. It would clearly be unfortunate if all this material were simply poured into the blood without some form of purification. This is where the lymph nodes come in. The nodes form a complex system of filters which remove or destroy most of the noxious material before it can enter the blood.

In principle, the nodes function by greatly widening the lymph channels so that the flow rate slows right down. The wide channels in the nodes are known as sinuses. Their effect is similar to the effect of a rapid river suddenly widening and slowing down as it enters a lake. All the sediment which the lymph has been carrying, such as cancer cells or bacteria, settles out. Much of this sediment is then engulfed by special cells which line the walls of the sinuses and are known as reticulo-endothelial or phagocytic cells. This is why, when a cancer or an infection develops in any part of the body, it tends to be temporarily stopped at the lymph nodes. In the case of infection, the nodes which receive the lymph draining from the infected area become swollen and painful. In the case of cancer, the growth develops in the nodes and may be prevented for some time from gaining entry to the blood.

The lymph which leaves the nodes is thus largely purified. The lymph channels come together and grow larger and eventually the lymphatic vessels pour lymph into the venous system at several sites. The most important one is via the thoracic duct which empties into the jugular vein at the side of the neck: this receives the lymph from most of the lower part of the body.

OEDEMA

Oedema is the word used to describe the excessive accumulation of fluid in the tissues. It has three main causes, each clearly related to one of the factors which govern the passage of fluid across the capillary wall.

1. *Capillary permeability.* If the capillary wall is damaged and becomes freely permeable to protein, then plasma proteins can no longer effectively exert an osmotic pressure. The blood pressure can thus act unopposed and fluid is lost rapidly from the capillaries: the fluid which is lost is effectively protein-rich plasma. Capillary damage happens particularly during burns and local infections.

2. *Raised pressure of capillary blood.* If the pressure of blood in the capillaries rises, then fluid will move out into the tissues more easily. Since capillary permeability is unchanged, the fluid lost has little or no protein in it. A rise in arterial pressure is usually not

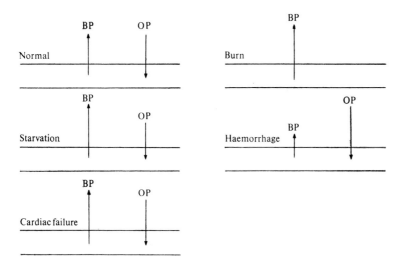

Fig.3.3. Imbalances between blood pressure and osmotic pressure which occur in various disease states.

transmitted to the capillaries because the arterioles constrict to prevent such transmission. In contrast, if venous pressure rises as it does in heart failure, the capillaries have no protection and the raised venous pressure is thus transmitted directly to them. This is why oedema is one of the outstanding features of heart failure.

3. *Plasma protein concentration.* If the concentration of plasma proteins falls, the osmotic pressure they exert also falls. The force drawing fluid into the blood is therefore reduced and fluid escapes from the capillaries more easily. This can occur in starvation and may help to account for the gross oedema sometimes seen in that condition.

4

The blood

The blood is the central means of transport within the body and it puts every organ in contact with every other organ. It has two main components, the plasma and the so-called 'formed elements'. The formed elements include:

1. Red cells, which contain the pigment haemoglobin which carries oxygen from the lungs to the tissues and carbon dioxide in the reverse direction.

2. White cells, which are primarily important in combating the invasion of foreign organisms and materials. They are much less numerous than the red cells.

3. Platelets, which are pale non-nucleated cell fragments manufactured by the cells known as megakaryocytes in the bone marrow. They are essential for the normal control of bleeding from a wound.

BLOOD VOLUME, HAEMATOCRIT AND RED CELL COUNT

The total blood volume in a normal adult is in the region of four to five litres, depending on size. The simplest way of roughly estimating the amount of red cells in a person is to take a small sample of blood, treat it with something to prevent clotting and to centrifuge it in a specially calibrated tube. The red cells settle out at the bottom of the tube. On top of them is an exceedingly thin layer of white cells which is sometimes known as 'the buffy coat'. Above the white cells is the clear, straw-coloured plasma. If the tube is calibrated it is easy to read off the percentages of red cells and plasma by volume: the volume of the white cells is well under 1 per cent of that of the whole blood. Usually about 45 per cent of the blood volume is made up of red cells and this is known as the haematocrit value.

The red cell count is the number of red blood cells in one cubic millimetre of blood. The count is usually in the region of 4·5 to 6 million/mm³. The count can be made manually using a microscope and special slide with a counting chamber, but increasingly automatic counting machines are coming into use.

ERYTHROCYTE SEDIMENTATION RATE (ESR)

The red blood cells are often known as erythrocytes. Because they are heavier than the plasma, if blood is treated with something to prevent it clotting and then simply left, the red cells will gradually settle out. This has been made the basis of the simple standard test of the erythrocyte sedimentation rate or ESR. The blood is drawn up into a narrow tube either 10 cm or 20 cm long depending on the precise technique being used. The tube is then left in the upright position for one hour and then the amount of clear plasma left above the red cells is noted. With a 20 cm tube, in normal young individuals the rate of fall is about 5 mm/hour. The ESR increases slowly with age, but rates over 15 mm/hour are probably always abnormal.

In disease the composition of the plasma proteins, and especially of the globulin component, changes as the body responds to the illness. For reasons which are still uncertain, these changes make the red cells more sticky and when they are left to stand they tend to come together in clumps. These clumps fall more rapidly than single red cells and so the sedimentation rate increases. In many diseases and particularly in cancer, coronary thrombosis and inflammatory conditions, the ESR is always high. If and as the patient gets better, the ESR gradually returns to normal.

The ESR is especially useful in two situations:

1. Many patients who consult doctors appear to be vaguely ill but it is impossible to diagnose their trouble with certainty. If the ESR is abnormally high, then there is certainly something wrong and the patient should be studied until it is found. A normal ESR does not exclude serious disease but it makes it unlikely.

2. Once a disease has been diagnosed and is being treated, the change in the ESR gives a rough indication of how the patient is progressing. If the ESR increases the patient is getting worse: if it decreases he is getting better.

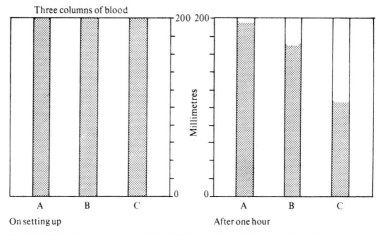

Three columns of blood

Fig.4.1. The determination of the ESR. Patient A is normal, patient B has a slightly raised ESR and patient C has a greatly raised ESR.

RED BLOOD CELLS (ERYTHROCYTES)

Both the red and the white cells are made in the bone marrow by the sequence of events shown in Fig.4.2. During fetal life the liver and spleen both take part in blood cell synthesis and may be able to do so again if during adult life the marrow is damaged. The red cells themselves are flat discs, squashed in a little in the centre of each side (biconcave). They normally live for about 120 days after leaving the marrow.

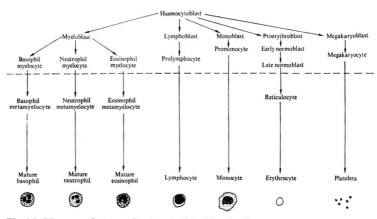

Fig.4.2. The manufacture of red and white blood cells.

The marrow in the bones is of two sorts, red and white. The red marrow is where red cell synthesis takes place. The white marrow mainly consists of fatty tissue, but like the liver and spleen it can begin to make red cells in an emergency. In adult life most of the red marrow is found in the bones of the skull, vertebral column, thorax and pelvis.

The rate at which the red cells are manufactured depends to a large extent on a hormone produced by the kidneys and known as erythropoietin. The existence of this hormone was first suggested by two clinical observations. In tumours of the kidneys excessive production of red cells frequently occurs, while in kidney failure severe anaemia (see next section) is very common. The hormone is at present relatively poorly understood. Its output is increased in anaemia in an effort to return the blood to normal and also during long exposure to low oxygen levels (as in mountain dwellers) when above normal amounts of haemoglobin are required to carry sufficient oxygen to the tissues.

The main function of the red cells is to carry haemoglobin, a red, iron-containing substance which is vital in the transport of oxygen and carbon dioxide around the body and in the maintenance of a steady blood pH. The normal range of haemoglobin concentration is 14–16 g/100 ml blood: women tend to be at the lower end of this range and men at the upper.

The haemoglobin molecule consists of two parts. There is a protein part known as globin and a non-protein, iron-containing part known as haem. As will be discussed later, each complete molecule of haemoglobin (Hb) is capable of combining with four molecules of oxygen.

When red cells become old, they are somehow identified as such and engulfed by the reticulo-endothelial (phagocytic) cells which line blood vessels in the liver, the bone marrow and the spleen. The protein is broken up, the iron is conserved for the manufacture of new red cells and the non-iron part of haem is converted to bilirubin, transported to the liver and excreted in the bile.

ANAEMIA AND NUTRITION

A person is said to be anaemic when the Hb concentration in the blood falls below normal. There are many causes of anaemia including blood parasites such as malaria, abnormalities of haemoglobin and chronic bleeding because of a peptic ulcer or heavy menstruation. Perhaps the most important cause, however, is a failure to take into the body basic materials required for the manufacture of red cells. Three factors are particularly important.

1. *Iron.* Iron deficiency anaemia is one of the commonest diseases in the world. If too little iron is taken in the food, too little Hb is made to fill the red cells normally. The red cells are therefore small (microcytic) and pale (hypochromic). Normal acid secretion by the stomach is necessary for the absorption of iron from the gut and in the absence of normal gastric function anaemia may occur.

2. *Folic acid.* This is a B group vitamin essential for the manufacture of the cells themselves but not so vital for the making of Hb. Folic acid deficiency therefore produces a shortage of cells and the red cell count is very low. The cells that are made tend to be larger than normal and carry more haemoglobin: they are sometimes known as macrocytes.

3. *Vitamin B_{12} (Cyanocobalamin).* This also is required for cell division and causes a macrocytic anaemia similar to that seen in folic acid deficiency. Anaemia due to vitamin B_{12} deficiency is often known as pernicious anaemia. Almost all diets, except those taken by extreme vegetarians, contain sufficient B_{12} and so a simple

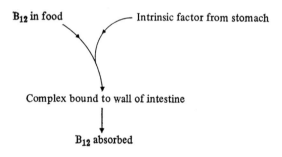

Fig.4.3. The absorption of vitamin B_{12}.

dietary deficiency is not the cause. However, B_{12} cannot be absorbed from the gut unless it first combines with a substance known as, intrinsic factor which is secreted by the stomach. If intrinsic factor is not secreted, even though there may be plenty of B_{12} in the diet, the vitamin goes straight through to the faeces without being significantly absorbed. Failure of normal intrinsic factor secretion is not uncommon. The disease can be cured by by-passing the gut altogether and giving the vitamin by means of regular injections. The absence of vitamin B_{12} also leads to damage to the spinal cord and peripheral nerves: it may cause behavioural changes. Folic acid deficiency does not cause these defects in functioning of the nervous system.

WHITE CELLS (LEUCOCYTES)

Most of the white cells are concerned with the body's reactions to injury and disease. When a pathologist is asked to look at the white cells in the blood, he usually does two things: he measures the total numbers in a known volume of blood (the normal white cell count is in the region of $5000–8000/mm^3$) and also measures the percentages of each type present (a differential white cell count). From measuring the total number and the percentages it is possible easily

Table 4.1. Approximate white cell concentrations and percentages in normal blood

	Percentage	*Concentration/mm³*
Neutrophils	50–70	3000–6000
Eosinophils	1–4	150–300
Basophils	0–1	0–100
Lymphocytes	20–40	1500–2700
Monocytes	2–8	300–600

to work out the numbers of each type. The main types of white cell are:

1. *Neutrophil polymorphs* (50–70 per cent). These are manufactured in the bone marrow. The name polymorph is short for 'polymorphonuclear' and indicates that the nucleus has a complex shape with a variable number of lobes. The word neutrophil indicates that they are stained by neutral dyes. About half the mature polymorphs in the body are not circulating freely in the blood but are stored in the lungs, spleen and marrow. Exercise and adrenaline (epinephrine) bring them out in large numbers as do infections and cell death of any kind, whether due to infection, cancer or injury. These conditions therefore all send the polymorph count soaring: a high count is a good indication that inflammation (for example, appendicitis) is taking place somewhere in the body. The neutrophil

polymorphs are continually being replaced and their normal life span is probably about five days. They are capable of actively ingesting foreign material and dead or dying body cells, by the process known as phagocytosis. Their main functions are therefore to combat bacterial invasion by eating the bacteria and to clear up the debris which results from cell damage. In any part of the body where infection or any other form of inflammation is occurring, the blood vessels become sticky. Neutrophils adhere to the sticky capillary walls and then push their way out through the walls into the interstitial fluid where they can operate to combat the disease process. In the course of this, many neutrophils are killed and dead neutrophils are a major component of the fluid known as pus.

2. *Eosinophil polymorphs* (normally 1–4 per cent). These have nuclei which are similar to those of the neutrophils. However, as their name implies eosinophils are stained red by acid dyes such as eosin and are not stained by neutral dyes. Their functions are not understood. Their numbers do not rise in acute infections and inflammations, but excessive numbers of eosinophils may be found in some chronic infections such as tuberculosis, in infestations with gut parasites such as worms and in allergic conditions like asthma and hay fever.

3. *Basophils*. These stain with basic dyes. Their function is again unknown but they are rich in histamine and the anti-clotting substance, heparin.

4. *Monocytes* (normally 2–8 per cent). These are relatively large cells with rounded nuclei. Like the neutrophil polymorphs they can engulf particles by means of phagocytosis. Also like the neutrophils they are attracted to places where infection and inflammation are occurring, but they usually appear on the scene rather later than the neutrophils. They live for several months and they clear up much of the debris left by the neutrophils. They particularly collect in places where foreign material stays in the body for a long time: surgical suture material and tuberculosis bacteria are examples of particles which tend to cause an accumulation of many monocytes. In such circumstances the monocytes often become transformed into giant cells with many nuclei.

5. *Lymphocytes* (normally 20–40 per cent). These are smallish cells with rounded nuclei and clear cytoplasm. They play a major part in the immune response and are discussed in the next section.

THE IMMUNE RESPONSE

Many types of foreign material, when they enter the body evoke what is known as an immune response. Substances which can evoke this response are usually protein in nature and are known as antigens. The response takes five to ten days to develop when a foreign antigen first gains access to the body. It has two main components.

1. *Cellular component.* This is particularly evident when the antigens are carried on the surfaces of foreign cells as in a transplanted organ. It depends on a type of lymphocyte which is able to migrate to the region where the foreign cells are found and their to destroy them by unknown means.

2. *Antibody component.* Some of the lymphocytes which come into contact with foreign antigens can become transformed into complex cells known as plasma cells, which are capable of manufacturing large amounts of a type of protein known as antibody. The antibody has the property of being able to combine with the antigen and so inactivating it. If the antigen is a chemical toxin such as that released by diphtheria bacteria, the combination with antibody can render the toxin non-poisonous. If the antigen is attached to a cell surface, the antigen-antibody combination may actually destroy the cell or make it much more susceptible to attack by neutrophils and monocytes.

There are two particularly remarkable features of the immune response. The first is that the response to each antigen is specific. Foreign antigen A will initiate immune response A with manufacture of antibody A: foreign antigen B will initiate immune response B with production of antibody B. Antibody B will not combine with antigen A and antibody A will not combine with antigen B. The second feature is that while the first time an antigen enters the body, the defence system takes several days to recognize it and to start the immune response, on the second occasion the response begins within a few hours. The defence system seems to 'remember' how to deal with an antigen it has met before. This explains why many diseases are caught only once: the second time exposure to infection occurs, the body is ready and waiting. It also explains the success of vaccination and immunization. The aim of these preventive measures is to expose the body to an antigen similar to one found on a disease-causing organism, but which is attached either to a living organism which is harmless or to a dead one. The body thus exposed to the antigen 'learns' about it and is able to mount a very rapid and effective immune response when faced with a real infection.

For cells capable of such complex activities, lymphocytes are surprisingly simple in appearance consisting of a round nucleus and a scanty amount of clear cytoplasm. They are made in the lymphoid tissue scattered throughout the body in the thymus gland, the gut wall, and the marrow, the spleen and the lymph nodes. The thymus gland, a rather ill-defined mass of tissue situated in the chest near the heart, and the gut lymphoid tissue appear to have particularly important roles in the development and the maintenance of the lymphocyte system. Although much remains to be understood, it seems probable that the thymus is primarily responsible for the lymphocytes which take part in the cellular part of the immune response, while the lymphoid tissue in the gut wall is responsible for the lymphocytes which can be transformed into plasma cells and produce antibody. Lymphoctyes gain entry to the circulatory system by entering the lymph vessels as they pass through lymph nodes and other types of lymphoid tissue. They are poured into the venous system, mostly via the thoracic duct. They leave the blood again via the capillaries in lymphoid tissue which have unusually permeable walls and thus recirculate continuously between blood and lymph.

PLASMA PROTEINS

Normal plasma contains 6–7 g of protein per 100 ml. There are two main types, the relatively low molecular weight albumins and the relatively high molecular weight globulins. It is now believed that most of the globulins are antibodies (immunoglobulins) formed in the course of immune responses.

The main function of the albumin seems to be to exert an osmotic pressure in order to maintain the fluid balance across the capillary wall. It may also combine with and so help to transport around the body bilirubin, fatty acids and some hormones.

By weight the globulins make up in the region of 40 per cent of the total amount of plasma protein. However, because globulin molecules are much larger than albumin ones, the globulins contribute less than 20 per cent to the total plasma protein osmotic pressure. Their prime importance is in immunity but some also have a role in the transport of metals, such as iron and copper, and of some hormones such as cortisol and thyroid hormone.

There are many other protein substances found in plasma but

their concentrations are low in comparison with albumins and globulins. They include:

1. Various clotting factors such as prothrombin (see later this chapter).

2. Plasminogen. This is an inactive substance which under appropriate conditions can be converted to active plasmin which can dissolve blood clots. As yet the details of the mechanism are obscure but much research is being done at the moment because of the importance of clots in the causation of heart disease and strokes.

3. Cholinesterase. This destroys acetyl choline. It also happens to destroy succinyl choline, a neuromuscular blocking agent which is widely used for producing brief paralysis during surgical operations. In one out of every two thousand or so people, the enzyme is congenitally absent. In normal life this seems to cause little difficulty, but such patients undergoing surgery may be paralysed for unusually long periods after the usual dose of succinyl choline.

BLOOD GROUPS

Suppose samples of blood are taken from a group of people, treated to prevent clotting, and then mixed together in pairs. With some pairs of blood samples nothing will happen but with other pairs the red cells will stick together in large clumps (agglutinate) and the cells themselves may be destroyed. Not until the early years of this century was the research done which explained this phenomenon. It was demonstrated that the human race could be divided into four categories according to the presence or absence of certain proteins on the surfaces of red cells and in the plasma. The red cell proteins are known as antigens or agglutinogens, while the proteins in the plasma are known as antibodies or agglutinins. The four categories are:

Group O. The red cells carry **NO** antigen but there are two antibodies, anti-A and anti-B in the plasma.

Group A. The red cells carry A antigen and there is anti-B antibody in the plasma.

Group B. The red cells carry B antigen and there is anti-A antibody in the plasma.

Group AB. The red cells carry both A and B antigens but the plasma contains neither anti-C nor anti-B antibodies.

4

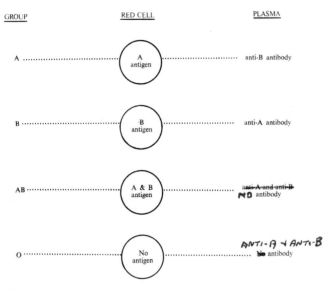

Fig.4.4. The red cells and plasma in the four main blood groups.

    The name of a person's group depends on the types of antigen found on his red cells. Whenever red cells carrying A antigen meet with anti-A antibody they will stick together and break up. Similarly whenever red cells carrying B antigen meet anti-B antibody they will stick together. The person's group can therefore be identified if one drop of his blood is mixed with a prepared serum containing anti-A antibody and another drop is mixed with a serum containing anti-B antibody. The mixing is usually done on a microscope slide and clumping together of red cells is looked for. The red cell group can then be readily identified by noting the results and consulting Table 4.2.

Table 4.2. Using this table it is possible by mixing red cells with Anti-A and with anti-B serum to determine the ABO group to which red cells belong. + means agglutination and can easily be seen because the agglutinated red cells clump together.

Cells	Anti-A serum	Anti-B serum
A	+	−
B	−	+
AB	+	+
O	−	−

When blood transfusions are given, it is very important that the two bloods from the patient receiving the blood and the patient giving it, should not react together. If the red cells do clump together they may be destroyed (haemolysed) releasing haemoglobin which may block small vessels, particularly in the kidneys and so cause renal failure. In the course of the reaction, chemicals known as pyrogens (chapter 11) which cause fever and shivering are often released.

When transfusing blood, samples of donor and recipient blood should always be mixed and observed before the transfusion takes place. This is the only certain way of ensuring that there will be no agglutination. In emergencies, this may not be possible and the following rules should then be observed:

1. If the recipient's ABO group is known, give blood of the same group.

2. If the recipient's blood group is unknown give group O (universal donor) blood. The O cells carry no antigens and therefore will not be agglutinated by the recipient's plasma even if it carries both anti-A and anti-B antibodies. The effect of the antibodies in the donor's plasma on the recipient's red cells can usually be ignored because they are so diluted by the recipient's plasma. This may not be true if the antibody concentration in the donor blood is unusually high or in cases where massive transfusion is required.

3. If the recipient's blood group is AB (universal recipient) then blood of any group can be given because there are neither anti-A nor anti-B antibodies in the recipient's plasma.

THE RHESUS PHENOMENON

In 1940 it was found almost by accident that an antibody against rhesus monkey red cells would agglutinate the red cells from most human beings. The human cells were agglutinated because they carried an antigen which became known as the rhesus (Rh) antigen. Those who carried the Rh antigen were known as Rh+. A small proportion of people (around 15 per cent) did not carry the Rh antigen on their red cells and were known as Rh−. It was soon realized that these findings might explain a not uncommon disease of new born infants. Infants with this disease, when they are born (and often before) suffer from excessive red cell destruction. They become very anaemic and the breakdown of large amounts of haemoglobin leads to jaundice. The bilirubin produced by this haemoglobin breakdown tends to accumulate in the brain and may cause permanent damage.

In each case when this happens, the baby and the father are Rh+ while the mother is Rh—. The baby inherits the Rh+ gene from its father. It is also known that the first Rh+ pregnancy in an Rh— women is almost never dangerous for the child, but that the risk tends to increase progressively with each succeeding pregnancy. In order to understand what is happening it is necessary to appreciate three facts in addition to those already presented.

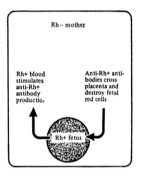

Fig.4.5. The mechanism of Rh disease.

1. During every pregnancy some cells from the baby's circulation enter the mother's blood. It is unusual for much of the baby's blood to enter the mother until labour begins. Then the uterine contractions inevitably force some of the baby's red cells into the mother's blood.

2. The Rh+ antigen is a foreign protein to an Rh— mother and so she mounts an immune response against it, in the course of which the cells carrying the antigen are destroyed. This immune response takes several days to develop fully.

3. The Rh blood group system differs from the ABO system in that an Rh— mother does not naturally have anti-Rh+ antibodies circulating in her blood.

It should now be possible to understand the following sequence of events, which occurs when an Rh— woman has several Rh+ children:

1. In the first pregnancy there are no anti-Rh+ antibodies in the mother's blood. During labour a significant quantity of Rh+ cells from the baby may enter the mother and stimulate the formation of anti-Rh+ antibodies. A few days later these antibodies destroy the baby's red cells present in the mother's circulation, but because the baby itself has gone they can have no effect on the child.

2. During a second Rh+ pregnancy the mother will already have been sensitized to the Rh+ antigen. On a second exposure, much smaller quantities of antigen are needed to provoke an immune response and the response occurs much more rapidly. Even if only a very few of the baby's red cells escape into the mother's circulation during the course of the pregnancy, they will stimulate an immediate immune response with the production of large amounts of anti-Rh+ antibody. This antibody may be produced well before the end of pregnancy.

3. If the mother's anti-Rh+ antibodies cross the placenta into the fetal circulation they will destroy the baby's red cells.

4. The baby will become anaemic and the large amounts of bilirubin produced may damage the brain. Brain damage is most likely to occur after birth because during the pregnancy the baby's bilirubin is effectively removed and excreted by the mother. But after birth the baby must rely entirely on its own liver for bilirubin excretion. Even in normal babies, for the first few days the liver may be unable to cope with the bilirubin produced by normal red cell destruction, giving the so-called 'physiological jaundice' which is common a few days after birth. In an Rh+ baby from an Rh− mother the situation is much worse.

The severity of rhesus haemolytic disease depends on the transfer of the baby's red cells to the mother and on the reverse transfer of the mother's anti-Rh+ antibodies to the baby. The degree to which these processes take place varies from pregnancy to pregnancy, accounting for the variation in intensity of Rh disease in different pregnancies in the same mother. Until recently all that could be done was to hope that the baby was not too affected and to give 'exchange transfusions' after birth to affected babies. In an exchange transfusion some of the baby's own blood is removed and an equal quantity of fresh donor blood is put back. This has the double effect of lowering the bilirubin levels and combating the anaemia. Recently two new techniques have considerably improved the outlook in Rh disease.

1. It is now possible to transfuse a baby even while it is still in the mother's uterus. Under X-ray control a needle is passed into the baby's peritoneal cavity and red cells are injected in. The red cells are, perhaps surprisingly, very rapidly absorbed into the blood stream.

2. The initial stage in Rh disease depends on the entry of the baby's red cells into the mother in significant amounts, usually at the time of the birth of the first Rh+ infant. If these red cells could be promptly destroyed, they would not be able to stimulate the mother's immune response and so sensitization could not occur. It has now been proved that the baby's red cells which appear in the mother can very rapidly be destroyed by injecting into the mother at the time of delivery anti-Rh+ antibodies. These rapidly haemolyse any fetal Rh+ cells and prevent the development of the immune response. By injecting anti-Rh+ antibody immediately after delivery in every pregnancy in an Rh− woman, it should be possible to prevent maternal sensitization almost entirely and so to eliminate rhesus disease in any population where reasonable standards of medical care are available to all.

BLOOD CLOTTING

As everyone knows, when blood is taken from a blood vessel and put into a container it does not remain liquid but clots. A normal clotting mechanism is obviously essential if the body is to respond to injury normally.

The sequence of events which occurs in clotting is very complex in detail but relatively simple in outline. Only the outline will be given here. The process may be started off in two ways:

1. If the blood comes into contact with an abnormal surface clotting may begin. An abnormal surface may arise in the body because of damage to blood vessel walls by injury, by infection, or as a result of oxygen lack which may occur when the blood in a vessel ceases to flow and becomes stagnant.

2. If products of damage to body tissues gain access to the blood the process of clotting is initiated. This may also occur during injury.

Both preliminary phases end up with the formation of a substance called thromboplastin (sometimes also known as active factor V).

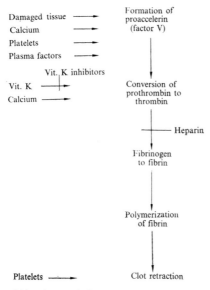

Fig.4.6. An outline of blood coagulation.

Calcium, and the non-nucleated formed elements of the blood known as platelets, are both essential for these preliminary stages leading to thromboplastin formation.

Thromboplastin is an enzyme which can act on a protein found in the blood known as prothrombin. Prothrombin is manufactured by the liver and vitamin K is essential for its synthesis. In the presence of calcium, thromboplastin converts prothrombin into another active enzyme known as thrombin. Thrombin then acts on another plasma protein, fibrinogen, to form fibrin. Fibrin consists of long threads which mesh together and trap red cells, white cells, platelets and plasma. The trapped platelets then release substances including serotonin or 5-hydroxytryptamine which cause the fibrin threads to contract, making the clot firmer and expelling the clear yellow fluid known as serum: this process is known as clot retraction. The difference between plasma and serum is often not understood. Plasma is the fluid part of the blood, excluding the formed elements: it can be obtained by centrifuging unclotted blood. Serum is identical to plasma apart from the fact that the clotting factors present in the plasma have been removed.

Nearly twenty factors have now been identified as being necessary for the normal clotting of blood and more seem to be discovered every year. Many diseases are known in which one of these factors is congenitally absent. The most famous is haemophilia due to absence of factor VIII or anti-haemophilic globulin. Haemophilia became famous because it is relatively common, because it occurred in some of the famous European royal families and because, since the normal gene is carried on the X chromosome and since females have two Xs but males only one, it is very much commoner in males than females. For a female to have haemophilia both her X chromosomes must be abnormal: females with one abnormal X chromosome do not show the disease, but they can pass on the abnormality and the disease to their sons. The main features of haemophilia and of most of the other clotting factor defects are a failure of wounds to stop bleeding and a tendency for bleeding to occur into joints. During normal exercise joint blood vessels often become damaged but the blood clots at once and causes no trouble. In haemophiliacs the bleeding from such minor injuries may continue for long periods.

When blood is withdrawn from one person in order to give a transfusion to another, it is obviously essential to stop the blood clotting in the bottle. This is usually done by withdrawing ionic calcium from the donor blood by means of a chemical reaction with citrate, oxalate or EDTA ('sequestrene'). Since free calcium ions are required for several stages in the coagulation process, these substances can effectively prevent clotting.

Anti-coagulants

The ease with which blood clots tends to be considerably increased after tissue damage such as occurs during a surgical operation or a heart attack. When patients are in bed, the blood in the leg veins tends to stagnate. The combination of these two factors may lead to abnormal and dangerous clotting within the blood vessels themselves. Such patients may therefore need treatment to reduce the clotting activity of the blood. They can be given two different types of drug.

1. *Heparin*. This was originally isolated from leeches which suck blood and which need to prevent it clotting so that they can feed properly. It is also found in the basophil leucocytes. It is digested by the human gut and so must be given by injection. It acts instantaneously, interfering with clotting by blocking the conversion of prothrombin to thrombin. Its action can be instantly reversed by

injecting the protein protamine which is found in fish sperm: the protamine acts by combining with the heparin.

2. *Oral anti-coagulant drugs.* There are many varieties of these, all acting by inhibiting the action of vitamin K in the liver. Some of the substances occur naturally in plants and can cause bleeding when eaten by farm animals. They prevent the manufacture of prothrombin and other clotting factors. They do not interfere with the actions of clotting factors already present in the blood, but as these factors are naturally used up and destroyed they are not replaced. The oral anti-coagulant drugs therefore take several days to act. When their intake is stopped the liver takes some time to restore the levels of clotting factors to normal.

HAEMOSTASIS

This is the stopping of bleeding from damaged blood vessels. It is often thought that clotting (coagulation) is the only process of importance in haemostasis, but this is not true. Even if clotting is defective, bleeding may stop entirely normally from small wounds of the skin: even if clotting is normal, other deficiencies may lead to prolonged bleeding from small wounds. The cessation of bleeding depends on three distinct but interlinked processes.

1. When small blood vessels are damaged, the injury stimulates the contraction of the muscular tissues in their walls. This muscle spasm tends to close off the vessel.

2. The damage stimulates platelets to stick together to form a plug over the hole which prevents the leakage of blood. This process is known as conglutination.

3. Finally the blood in the damaged vessel clots to form a firm plug which will control the escape of blood until healing has taken place.

With small wounds the first two processes alone may be able to stop bleeding, but with large wounds haemostasis cannot occur unless clotting is normal.

THE SPLEEN

Although most people can survive entirely satisfactorily without a spleen, the organ nevertheless does perform important functions.

It is rich in lymphoid tissue. It contains blood sinuses which are lined by phagocytic reticulo-endothelial cells which can engulf particles from the blood.

The main functions of the spleen are:

1. Red cell manufacture occurs in the spleen in the fetus. In children or adults whose bone marrow has been damaged or destroyed, the spleen may start making red cells again.

2. Removal of unwanted particles from the blood. The spleen is important in the destruction of ageing red and white cells and platelets.

3. The lymphoid tissue like lymphoid tissue everywhere plays an important part in the immune response.

4. Red cell storage. This is known to be of importance in carnivorous animals. To meet an emergency the spleen contracts vigorously pouring out a large store of red cells held within the sinuses into the general circulation. The importance of this is not known in man.

5

Circulation

The circulation forms the body's transport system which by pumping blood puts every part of the body in communication with every other part. First it is important to have an outline of the structure of the system.

The human heart contains four chambers. Blood from the peripheral areas of the body apart from the lungs is returned by the veins to the thin-walled right atrium. From there it passes to the right ventricle which pumps it out along the pulmonary artery to the lungs where it is oxygenated. The pulmonary veins return the oxygenated blood to the left atrium from which it passes into the left ventricle which pumps it out into the aorta and so to the peripheral parts of the body. The period when the heart is contracting and pumping blood out is known as systole and the period when it is relaxing and letting blood in is known as diastole. The heart is an effective pump because the entries to and exits from the ventricles are controlled by non-return valves. When the ventricles contract the valves guarding the channel between the atria and ventricles

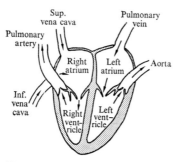

Fig.5.1. An outline of heart structure.

(tricuspid valve on the right and mitral valve on the left) close to prevent any backward flow of blood. The valves controlling the exits from the ventricles to the pulmonary artery on the right and aorta on the left, open to let the blood out. The valve in the pulmonary artery is known as the pulmonary valve and the one in the aorta as the aortic valve.

As it passes round the body, the blood first goes through arteries, then arterioles, then capillaries, then venules and then veins before getting back to the heart again. All the blood vessels except the capillaries have four layers in their walls:

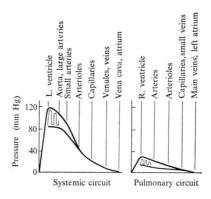

Fig.5.2. The pressures in the various blood vessels in a normal individual.

1. An innermost lining of endothelial cells, one cell thick. This layer is the only one present in the capillaries. It allows all the constituents of the blood except the cells and plasma proteins to pass through it freely and it is therefore in the capillaries that the exchange between blood and tissues take place. The other three layers are relatively impermeable to the passage of plasma and its constituents.

2. An inner layer of connective tissue fibres, mainly arranged longitudinally.

3. A middle layer of mixed connective and muscle fibres (tunica media) arranged circularly.

4. An outer layer of connective tissue fibres arranged irregularly (tunica adventitia).

Both elastin fibres (which stretch more easily than rubber) and collagen fibres (which are resistant to stretch) are found in the connective tissue.

In arteries all three outer layers are well-developed but the middle layer contains much more elastic tissue than muscular tissue. As the arteries divide and decrease in diameter, the inner and outer layers of connective tissue become much thinner and the proportion of muscle in the middle layer increases giving the vessels known as arterioles. The arterioles give way to the capillaries, an intricate network of minute vessels with walls only one cell thick. The capillaries coalesce to give venules which in turn combine to give

Table 5.1. The measurements of the blood vessels to the gut in the dog showing the changes in size and number of vessels at different levels.

Vessel	Diameter (mm)	Number	Total cross-sectional area (cm²)
Aorta	10	1	0·8
Main arterial branches	1	600	5·0
Arterioles	0·02	40 million	125
Capillaries	0·008	1200 million	600
Main venous branches	2·4	600	27
Vena cava	12·5	1	1·2

veins which have much thinner walls than the corresponding arteries. Table 5.1. gives some information about the number, diameter, cross sectional area and volume of the blood vessels in the gut of a mammal. It is important to note that although the capillaries are so small, there are so many of them that their total cross sectional area in this single vascular bed is about six hundred times that of the aorta.

The muscle pump

The heart is not the only pump in the body. The veins also contain no-return valves. If a vein is compressed by muscular activity the blood is squeezed out and has no alternative but to move towards the heart. At rest the muscle pump is ineffective and all the work of pumping the blood around the body must be done by the heart. But during exercise when the muscles are repeatedly contracting and relaxing, quite a high proportion of the work of the circulation may be carried out by this muscle pump.

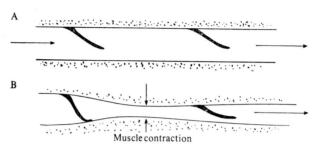

A

B

Muscle contraction

Fig.5.3. The valves in the veins mean that when the vessel is compressed the blood must be pumped on towards the heart. A Rest. B. Contraction.

HEART MUSCLE

When seen under a microscope heart muscle appears to be striated but it differs in several ways from skeletal muscle. It consists of branching fibres which are extremely closely attached to one another by structures known as intercalated discs. The effect is to link all the fibres very closely together both structurally and functionally. In behaviour heart muscle differs in two major ways from skeletal muscle.

Intercalated disc

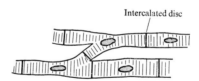

Fig.5.4. Heart muscle fibres.

1. It has a very long refractory period which lasts longer than the period of contraction. In skeletal muscle the refractory period lasts not much more than 0·001 sec. while the contraction lasts from 0·2–0·5 sec. This means that if two nerve impulses follow one another very quickly the muscle has no time to relax and the contractions add on to one another. It would be quite disastrous if this sort of thing happened with the heart. The heart depends for its action on a strong contraction which pumps out the blood and which is always followed by a period of relaxation when the heart can fill with blood again ready for the next contraction. It is essential that contractions should not be able to follow one another too quickly: this is achieved

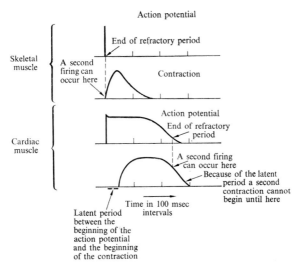

Fig.5.5. A comparison of the action potentials and subsequent contractions in skeletal and cardiac muscle. In skeletal muscle there is virtually no latent period between the action potential and the beginning of the contraction but in cardiac muscle the latent period is relatively long.

by the very long refractory period, longer than the contraction itself, which ensures that the muscle cannot be excited again until it has fully relaxed.

2. Even in the total absence of nerves, heart muscle strips contract spontaneously and rhythmically. Skeletal muscle normally contracts only in response to a nervous impulse: in the absence of such an impulse it remains relaxed. But even if all the nerves to the heart are cut, or even if strips of heart muscle are bathed in an appropriate oxygenated solution, the heart muscle fibres contract spontaneously in a rhythmic manner. The use of isolated strips taken from different parts of the heart, reveals that heart muscle may be divided into three broad categories according to its origin and behaviour.

a. Muscle from the so-called 'pacemaker region' (the area in the right atrium known as the sino-atrial or SA node) beats fastest with a spontaneous rate of about 70–80 beats per minute.

b. Muscle from other parts of the atria beats spontaneously at about 50–70 beats per minute.

c. Muscle from the ventricles beats slowest at a natural rate of 20–40 beats per minute.

CONDUCTION OF THE CARDIAC IMPULSE

As in skeletal muscle, contraction of cardiac muscle is fired off by an impulse (action potential) spreading over the surfaces of the muscle fibres. In skeletal muscle, the muscle impulse must be fired off by a nerve impulse reaching the neuromuscular junction. In cardiac muscle the muscle impulse arises spontaneously without nervous action.

There is a group of muscle fibres in the right atrium known as the sino-atrial (SA) node. The SA node is sometimes called the pacemaker since its fibres naturally beat faster than other heart muscle

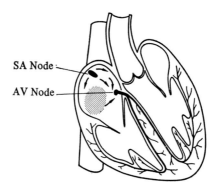

SA Node

AV Node

Fig.5.6. The conducting system of the heart.

fibres and because it 'calls the tune' forcing the other parts of the heart to follow its rhythm under normal circumstances.

When an impulse arises spontaneously in the SA node it spreads out along the atrial muscle fibres so making the atria contract. The atria and the ventricles are almost completely separated from one another by fibrous connective tissue which does not conduct impulses. The only conducting connection between the atria and ventricles is a small piece of specialized muscle tissue known as the atrio-ventricular (AV) node. Here the conducting fibres become very thin and in consequence the impulse travels very slowly from the atria to the ventricles. This ensures that the contraction of the atria is virtually completed by the time the impulse reaches the ventricles.

On the ventricular side there is a specialized system of muscle fibres known as Purkinje fibres which conduct the impulse extremely rapidly to all parts of the ventricle. They are first gathered together in the bundle of His, but this soon divides into right and left bundle branches which go to their respective ventricles. The Purkinje fibres do conduct the impulse rapidly so that it arrives almost simultaneously at all parts of the ventricles. This enables all the ventricular fibres to contract vigorously together.

THE HEART RATE

The natural spontaneous rate of beating of the pacemaker may be altered in four main ways:

1. Sympathetic nerves to the SA node release noradrenaline which increases the rate of beating.

2. Vagal (parasympathetic) fibres to the SA node release acetyl choline which slows down the rate of beating.

3. Circulating adrenaline which has been released from the adrenal medulla acts on the SA node to increase the heart rate.

4. Distension of the right atrium due to overfilling with blood causes the SA node fibres to be stretched and this makes them contract more vigorously. This may be one of the factors which helps to account for the fast heart rate in the condition known as congestive cardiac failure when the heart is greatly dilated.

THE CARDIAC CYCLE

The action of the heart can be conveniently divided into four phases. The description which follows applies to the left side of the heart but the right side behaves in a similar manner.

1. As the ventricle relaxes after its last beat, the pressure of blood within it falls rapidly. When the pressure in the ventricle becomes lower than that in the atrium the mitral valve opens and blood rushes in to the empty ventricle. As the ventricle becomes full, the rate of filling slows down. It receives a boost when the atrium contracts so forcing a little extra blood into the ventricle. It should be noted, however, that the ventricles can fill reasonably well even in the absence of atrial contraction.

2. Because of the delay at the AV node, the ventricle contracts well after the atrium. As soon as the ventricular contraction begins, the pressure of the blood in the ventricle rises sharply. As soon as the

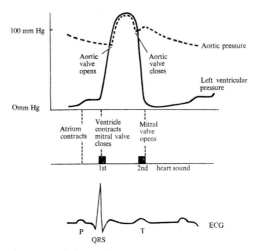

Fig.5.7. The main events of the cardiac cycle.

pressure in the ventricle becomes higher than the pressure in the atrium the mitral valve closes. As pressure rises higher, the pressure in the ventricle becomes higher than the pressure in the aorta and this forces open the aortic valves. Blood rushes out into the aorta. When a person is resting, the ventricle pumps out only about half the blood it contains, the remainder staying in the ventricle at the end of the beat. During exercise the ventricle beats more vigorously and less blood is left behind at the end of each beat.

3. As the ventricle relaxes, pressure inside it falls below the pressure in the aorta. When this happens the aortic valve snaps shut, so preventing any backflow from the aorta into the heart. As relaxation continues, pressure in the ventricle falls below that in the atrium. The mitral valve opens to let the blood which has been accumulating in the atrium flow into the ventricle.

THE HEART SOUNDS

When you use a stethoscope to examine the cardiovascular system, two forms of sound can be heard:

1. The classical heart sounds originate as vibrations in various parts of the heart, notably the valves.

2. Sounds may arise in the heart or in any of the large vessels due

to the turbulent flow of blood. These sounds are softer than the classical heart sounds and are commonly known as murmurs.

Two heart sounds can be clearly heard in any normal person by anyone who picks up a stethoscope for the first time. They are often described as sounding like lub-dup. The first sound is due to the closing of the mitral and tricuspid valves: the closing of the two is normally synchronous and only one sound can be heard. The second sound is due to the closure of the aortic and pulmonary valves. These events may be synchronous or, even in healthy people, the second sound may be slightly split because the contraction of the left ventricle is completed a fraction of a second before that of the right. It is thus apparent that the period between lub and dup corresponds to the period of ventricular contraction (systole) while the period between dup and lub corresponds to ventricular relaxation (diastole).

In addition to the heart sounds various murmurs due to turbulent flow of blood may arise in the heart:

1. Those occurring between the first sound (lub) and the second sound (dup) arise during ventricular contraction and must therefore be associated with the turbulent expulsion of blood from the ventricle.

   a. If the tricuspid or mitral valves fail to close properly (valvular incompetence) there may be an abnormal backward flow of blood from ventricle to atrium.

   b. Turbulence may simply be caused by a very rapid flow of blood through normal aortic valves. This may occur in the smaller vessels of children, especially during exercise, and has no pathological significance.

   c. The pulmonary or aortic valves may fail to open properly (valvular stenosis). Turbulence occurs as the blood is forced out through the abnormally narrow opening.

2. Murmurs occurring between the second and first sounds, during ventricular relaxation, must be associated with the flow of blood into the ventricles.

   a. If the aortic or pulmonary valves are incompetent they may not close properly and backward flow from the pulmonary artery or aorta into the ventricles may occur.

   b. Stenosis of the tricuspid or mitral valve may cause a murmur as blood flows through the narrowed channel.

THE ELECTROCARDIOGRAM (ECG OR EKG)

When the heart muscle contracts, it sets up small electrical currents which are conducted through the body fluids. These currents may be detected by electrodes connected to the skin at appropriate points and connected to a sensitive recording instrument known as an electrocardiograph. The electrodes may be attached to the arms and legs and to the chest. By recording from different parts of the body the contribution made by the activity of different parts of the heart may be emphasized.

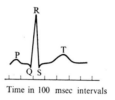

Time in 100 msec intervals

Fig.5.8. A normal ECG from lead II.

A normal ECG from 'lead II' (electrodes on the right arm and left leg) is shown in Fig.5.8. Five waves are conventionally described. The P wave is associated with the contraction of the atrial muscle fibres. The Q, R and S waves occur very close together and are often known as the QRS complex. They are associated with the start of ventricular muscle contraction. The T wave is associated with the end of ventricular contraction.

As a result of long experience, changes in the ECG pattern have come to be associated with particular cardiovascular diseases such as coronary thrombosis and hypertension. The ECG is therefore now a very important technique in diagnosis.

ARRHYTHMIAS

When the heart is beating entirely normally it is sometimes said to be in sinus rhythm because it is following the rhythm set by the sino-atrial node. Deviations from this normal rhythm are called arrhythmias. There are many varieties but some of the more important ones are as follows:

1. *Ectopic beats.* These are additional beats occurring outside the normal rhythm. They may arise anywhere in the heart, either in the atria or the ventricles because of some unusual irritability of part of the muscle. They may be of no pathological significance or they may indicate serious disease.

2. *Atrial flutter.* The atrial contractions are regular, but very rapid (often over 200 per minute). Since the refractory period of ventricular muscle is longer than that of atrial muscle, the ventricles cannot contract more than about 200 times per minute. This means that some of the atrial impulses arrive at the AV node while the ventricle is refractory. The ventricle usually beats relatively regularly but one in every two, three or four of the atrial impulses fails to get through.

3. *Atrial fibrillation.* The rate of beating of the atrial fibres is extremely rapid (often over 400 per minute) and is no longer regular. The AV node is therefore bombarded with hundreds of irregular impulses every minute. Only a few get through and the ventricular beat is very irregular. Relatively common causes of atrial fibrillation are stenosis of the mitral valve and overactivity of the thyroid gland although the precise mechanisms are not well understood. Perhaps surprisingly, neither atrial flutter nor atrial fibrillation reduce the cardiac output to levels which are immediately dangerous.

4. *Ventricular fibrillation.* The ventricular muscle fibres beat very rapidly and in a totally uncoordinated way so that the ventricle as a whole cannot contract. The patient dies quickly because cardiac pumping falls to zero unless defibrillation is brought about rapidly. This may sometimes be achieved by giving the patient a sharp blow on the chest. More usually it is necessary to give a strong electric shock to the heart through special electrodes. This causes all the heart muscle fibres to contract simultaneously and subsequently to become refractory simultaneously. On recovery from the refractory state the heart may begin to beat normally. The commonest cause of ventricular fibrillation is probably coronary thrombosis, but excessive amounts of adrenaline can sometimes initiate it, especially in patients who are anaesthetized.

5. *Heart block.* There are many types of damage to the conducting system. The simplest to understand is complete heart block in which the AV node ceases to function. The atria continue to beat at their normal rate of about 70 per minute, but no impulses can get through to the ventricles which therefore beat at their normal isolated rate of arou nd 30 per minute.

IONS AND THE HEART

If the heart is to beat normally, the blood passing through it must contain precisely the right concentration of certain ions and in particular of potassium and calcium.

Raising the potassium concentration weakens contractions and may cause arrhythmias or even stop the heart. Lowering the potassium concentration makes the heart abnormally excitable and may also cause arrhythmias. A high potassium concentration tends to occur in renal failure when the kidneys cannot excrete potassium ions normally. Low potassium concentrations are most common in patients who are being treated with diuretics to increase urine flow, for many diuretics increase urinary potassium loss. Low potassium levels are particularly dangerous in the presence of digitalis and when the two are present together arrhythmias occur frequently.

High concentrations of calcium can stop the heart in systole. This could occur during overactivity of the parathyroid glands when there is excessive loss of calcium from the bones into the blood, but in practice is uncommon.

THE PULSE

When the left ventricle pumps blood out, the blood initially enters the aorta far more rapidly than it can leave via the major arteries. The aorta therefore stretches in order to accommodate the extra blood. During diastole, as the blood flows away, the aorta returns to its normal size. This stretching sets up a pulse wave in the arterial walls: this wave has nothing to do with the actual flow of blood along the arteries and travels much more rapidly. The speed of travel of the pulse wave increases as the arterial walls become stiffer with advancing age. In childhood it travels at about 4 m/sec and in old age at about 10 m/sec.

The pressure difference between the peak pressure reached in the aorta during systole and the lowest pressure during diastole is known as the pulse pressure. The greater this pressure the more powerful will be the wave set up and the stronger the pulse will feel. The following are some important factors which alter the strength of the pulse:

1. The amount of blood ejected by the ventricle in one beat (the stroke volume). The more blood is pumped out, the greater will be the pressure rise and the stronger will be the pulse.

2. The stiffness of the aorta. The stiffer the aorta, the greater will be the pressure rise and the stronger will be the pulse.

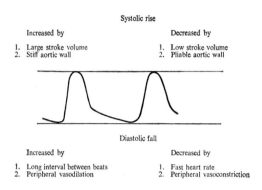

Systolic rise

Increased by
1. Large stroke volume
2. Stiff aortic wall

Decreased by
1. Low stroke volume
2. Pliable aortic wall

Diastolic fall

Increased by
1. Long interval between beats
2. Peripheral vasodilation

Decreased by
1. Fast heart rate
2. Peripheral vasoconstriction

Fig.5.9. Factors which affect the pulse pressure.

3. The rate of outflow from the aorta. Blood may leave the aorta rapidly if the aortic valve is incompetent so allowing blood to pass back into the ventricle, or if the peripheral arterioles are open wide so that blood can flow into the capillaries very rapidly. This rapid outflow of blood will lower the diastolic pressure and increase the pulse pressure. If there is marked vasoconstriction of the arterioles such as may occur after a haemorrhage, the rate of outflow from the aorta will be reduced and the pulse pressure will be low.

4. The rate of beating of the heart. The faster the heart is beating, the less chance is there for pressure to fall between beats and the lower will be the pulse pressure.

THE BLOOD PRESSURE

Undoubtedly the most accurate way to measure arterial pressure is to stick a needle connected to a sensing device into a major artery. For most purposes this is impractical and an indirect instrument, the sphygmomanometer must be used.

A wide rubber bag is wrapped around the upper arm at about the level of the heart. The rubber bag is connected to a manometer for measuring the pressure within it and to a simple pump by which it can be inflated. Before the bag is blown up, the brachial artery is detected at the elbow by palpitation and the stethoscope bell is placed over it. Nothing can be heard because the flow in the artery is smooth and laminar and not turbulent. The bag is then blown up to a pressure of around 250 mm Hg which is well above the systolic pressure in most individuals. This high pressure will stop blood flowing through the brachial artery since it is well above the systolic pressure in most individuals: no sounds can be heard through the stethoscope. While listening through the stethoscope, the pressure in the bag is then slowly released by means of a valve. Most people can hear three types of sound:

1. When the bag pressure falls just below the systolic pressure, a spurt of blood will force open the artery for a moment as the pressure in the artery reaches its peak. The spurt of blood causes rapid, turbulent flow and a sharp tapping sound occurs each time the ventricle ejects blood into the aorta.

2. As long as the bag pressure is above the diastolic pressure, the artery will be closed during each diastolic period when the pressure within it falls. When the bag pressure falls just below diastolic pressure, blood will flow through the artery during diastole as well as systole. The sounds then become less clear and distinct and tend to run into one another. This change is known as muffling.

3. The bag may partially block the artery during diastole until much lower pressures are reached. This may cause turbulence of flow and a sound which does not disappear until the bag pressure falls much lower.

It is widely agreed that the appearance of the sharp tapping sound is a good indication of the true systolic pressure. There is not nearly so much agreement about what indicates the diastolic pressure: some authorities think that the muffling indicates diastolic pressure while others use the disappearance of sounds. Fortunately the muffling and disappearance occur quite close together in most people and for practical purposes either one can be used, provided that it is used consistently.

THE CARDIAC OUTPUT

The cardiac output may be defined as the volume of blood pumped out by the left ventricle in one minute. It depends on the rate of the heart (the number of beats/min) and on the stroke volume (the amount of blood pumped out in one beat).

In a normal adult the cardiac output is usually in the region of 4–5 litres/min. In exercise it may increase enormously to 30 litres/min

Table 5.2. Approximate distribution of the cardiac output at rest. During exercise kidney and gut flow are greatly decreased and muscle flow is greatly increased

Kidney	20–25%
Liver and gut	30–35%
Muscle	10–20%
Head	15–20%
Heart	3– 7%
Other organs	10–20%

or more. In a resting person the actual distribution of the blood to the various organs of the body is shown in Table 5.2. During exercise the blood flow to the gut and to the kidneys is cut down considerably and more blood is diverted to the working muscles.

The cardiac output may be altered by changing either the heart rate or the stroke volume, or both simultaneously. The ways in which the heart rate may be changed have already been mentioned earlier in this chapter. Here we shall be concerned with stroke volume.

It is important to realize that in a normal resting individual the ventricles do not normally push out with each beat all the blood that they contain. If a ventricle contains 80 ml of blood at the end of the filling phase and before contraction begins, only 40–50 ml may be pumped out with each beat leaving 30–40 ml of blood behind. There are two main ways in which the stroke volume may be altered:

1. The maximum heart size during the cardiac cycle (i.e. the heart size when the ventricles are full just before contraction begins) may remain unchanged but the ventricles may beat more vigorously during each systole. This means that a greater proportion of blood is pumped out. In the terms of the example just given, the left ventricle may still contain only 80 ml when filling has been completed, but instead of pumping out 40–50 ml, it will pump out 60–80 ml. The ventricles may be made to beat more vigorously in two main ways:

   a. By the action of noradrenaline released from the sympathetic nerves to the heart.

   b. By the action of adrenaline released from the adrenal medulla into the circulating blood.

2. When stretched up to a certain limit, all types of muscle contract more vigorously than when they are not stretched. If the stretching goes beyond the limit, however, the ability of the muscle to contract fails rapidly. Heart muscle is no exception to this general rule and if the ventricles become stretched because they contain a larger amount of blood at the end of the filling phase they will contract more vigorously. This mechanism is important in two main situations:

   a. At the beginning of exercise when many of the skeletal muscles start contracting, blood is squeezed out of the veins because of the muscle pump. This means that there is a sudden increase in the venous return of blood to the right heart. This may temporarily stretch the right ventricle and make it contract more vigorously.

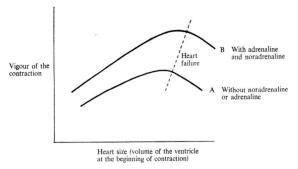

Fig.5.10. The relationship between the size of the heart (the stretch of the heart muscle fibres) and the amount of work it can do.

   b. When a heart is failing for any reason, it can no longer pump out the normal amount of blood so easily. This means that more blood tends to be left in the ventricles at the end of systole. During diastole a normal amount of blood comes back from the heart to fill the ventricles and the result is that at the end of the filling phase the ventricles contain more blood than normal. The heart as a whole becomes fuller and larger than it was before. The stretch of the ventricular muscle temporarily restores the ability of the heart to pump out a normal stroke volume. As the heart progressively fails it therefore becomes bigger and bigger (because it contains more blood at the end of the filling phase) in an effort to pump out a bigger stroke volume. The stretching continues until the limit is reached where further stretching causes a decrease in contractile vigour rather than an increase. When this point is reached, unless effective treatment is carried out there is a rapid decline in cardiac output and the person tends to die.

THE PERIPHERAL CIRCULATION

Once the blood leaves the left ventricle it is carried to the tissues by arteries, arterioles and capillaries. On leaving the capillaries it is taken back to the right heart by the venules and veins. All these vessels constitute what is known as the peripheral circulation.

Arteries

These are tough walled tubes whose main function is simply to act as conduits through which the blood is carried to the tissues. Their walls are rich in elastic and muscular tissue and this makes them very strong. If an artery is cut, the muscle in its wall contracts very vigorously and this contraction may even succeed in closing quite a large vessel.

Arterioles

The function of the arteries is simply to act as channels carrying blood to the organs. They do not regulate the amount of blood going to a particular organ and they are not under minute by minute control by nerves or hormones. The arterioles are quite different. They are formed as a result of the repeated branching of arteries and they are small vessels very rich in smooth muscle. This smooth muscle can be controlled by nerves, by hormones and by some other chemicals. It can contract to narrow the arterioles which supply blood to an organ so greatly reducing the blood flow. On the other hand the muscle can relax, so opening the arterioles wide and allowing large amounts of blood to flow into a tissue. The main ways in which the behaviour of the arteriolar smooth muscle can be controlled are:

1. Sympathetic nerves which release noradrenaline (norepinephrine). These go to all the arterioles in the body and the noradrenaline which they release causes constriction of the vessels. In the 'resting' state, the sympathetic nerves are moderately active

so that the vessels are neither wide open nor tightly shut. If the number of impulses passing down the nerves is increased, more noradrenaline is released and the arterioles close further. If the impulse activity is reduced, the smooth muscle can relax and the arterioles open wide (dilate).

2. Adrenaline (epinephrine) released from the adrenal medulla during exercise, fear, anger and other emergencies. Adrenaline differs from noradrenaline in that it has a dual action. It strongly constricts most of the arterioles in the body, apart from those in the muscles and the heart which it dilates. This is because while most arterioles are dominated by α receptors, those in the muscles and heart are dominated by β receptors. The overall action of adrenaline is therefore to reduce the flow of blood to organs like the skin, gut and kidneys which are not urgently needed in emergency situations and to increase blood flow to the muscles and heart which do need the extra blood.

3. Chemicals. Oxygen lack, carbon dioxide excess and excess of acid all tend to cause dilatation of arterioles, particularly in muscle, in the brain and in the heart. If the oxygen content of the blood falls, if its carbon dioxide content rises and if excess acids are being produced, these are indications that the tissues are not getting enough blood. It therefore makes sense that such chemical stimuli should dilate the arterioles in order to increase the flow of blood to a tissue.

Many other chemicals and hormones can alter the behaviour of arterioles but in most cases we do not yet understand their significance and so they will not be further considered here.

Capillaries

The capillaries, which have walls only one cell thick, are the smallest vessels in the body. Only in the capillaries can exchange of materials take place between the blood and the tissues: in all other blood vessels the relatively thick walls prevent such exchange occurring. In the capillaries there is a delicate balance between the blood pressure pushing fluid out and the osmotic pressure of the plasma proteins pulling fluid back (see chapter 3 on body fluids). The blood pressure tends to be slightly higher than the osmotic pressure at the beginning of a capillary and so fluid tends to leave the vessel there. By the end of the capillary, the pressure of the blood has fallen while the osmotic pressure of the plasma proteins is virtually unchanged: this means that the plasma protein osmotic pressure is usually higher than the blood pressure and so fluid is drawn back into the vessels. There is often a slight excess of outward over inward movement of fluid and this excess is drained away from the tissues in the form of lymph.

Venules and veins

The capillaries run together to form tiny vessels which are sometimes called venules and the venules run together to form veins. The veins have thin but relatively muscular walls and under normal conditions they contain about 60 per cent of all the blood in the vascular system. The muscles in the vein walls are controlled by sympathetic nerve fibres and when they contract they can push a surprisingly large volume of blood out of the veins and towards the heart. On the other hand if the smooth muscle in the veins relaxes completely and the vessels dilate fully, the venous system may be capable of holding 90 per cent of all the blood in the circulatory system.

All the veins except the very largest ones have valves. These are important because they prevent the pressure due to the whole column of venous blood being transmitted down the veins to the feet. If the valves are not functioning properly, the leg veins are subjected to a high pressure and become tortuous and dilated (varicose veins). The high pressure is also transmitted to the capillaries and excess fluid escapes from the blood in the lower part of the legs and the feet and oedema results.

The valves are particularly important during exercise. Because they do not allow the blood to flow backwards, when the veins are compressed by the muscles the blood must flow on towards the heart, thus helping the circulation. Normally in the legs the valves allow blood to flow only from the superficial veins into the deep veins of the muscles. If the valves of these so-called perforating vessels are not functioning, during exercise venous blood at high pressure is forced out of the muscles back into the superficial veins. This back flow is an important factor in the causation of varicose veins.

CIRCULATION THROUGH SPECIAL REGIONS

Many of the individual organs have peculiarities about the way in which the blood flow through them is controlled. Some of the most important organs are briefly considered in this section.

The brain

The nervous control of brain blood vessels is ineffective. Instead, the dilatation and constriction of the arterioles is determined almost entirely by the local chemical conditions. The most powerful stimulus for opening up the cerebral arterioles is an accumulation of carbon dioxide which indicates that not enough blood is reaching that part of the brain. Oxygen lack also has a strong dilating action. Blood flow through the brain thus depends almost entirely on local conditions. The brain demands and usually receives the blood flow it requires irrespective of what is happening elsewhere in the body.

The heart

Circulation through the heart too is controlled almost entirely by local chemical factors, although circulating adrenaline is a strong dilator. Oxygen lack is the most important stimulus, carbon dioxide accumulation being rather less important than in the brain. Again the heart demands blood, irrespective of what it is happening elsewhere.

Skeletal muscles

In the muscles nervous control by sympathetic fibres, circulating adrenaline and local chemical factors are all important. During rest, the blood flow through the muscles is very low indeed. However, when exercise begins and the muscles contract, oxygen is quickly used up and carbon dioxide and acids accumulate. These cause arteriolar dilatation, which is accentuated by the action of circulating adrenaline from the adrenal medulla.

The skin

The skin is an organ which, at least in the short term, is not vital to life and which primarily acts as the servant of the rest of the body, particularly in the regulation of body temperature. Because of this, sympathetic nervous control of the skin arterioles is very powerful: it regulates skin blood flow in accordance with the needs of the rest of the body, often over-riding the local requirements of the skin. When the body is cold, skin blood flow is cut to the minimum to reduce the loss of heat. When the body is warm, the skin circulation is opened up in order to increase the rate of heat loss. Only when the skin is in actual danger of either freezing or burning do local factors tend to predominate: in both cases skin blood flow increases in order to reduce the risk of damage.

The gut

In the gut, too, nervous control by noradrenaline released by the sympathetic system is very strong. When the gut is full of food, the vessels are open wide in order to allow plenty of blood to flow in for digestion. During exercise or any other emergency, however, the arterioles constrict and gut blood flow is cut to the bare minimum, the blood being diverted to tissues where it is urgently needed. This is why it is not advisable to take vigorous exercise soon after a meal: the blood is diverted from the gut and so digestion is delayed.

The kidneys

In order to carry out their functions the kidneys require a very high blood flow for most of the day. They normally receive about 25 per cent of the cardiac output. However, in emergency situations such as haemorrhage and exercise, the blood is diverted from the kidneys to organs which are more immediately vital and so in these circumstances the flow of urine may be considerably reduced.

THE CONTROL OF BLOOD PRESSURE

If the cardiovascular system is to function satisfactorily, the pressure within the arteries must be neither too high nor too low. It must be sufficient to push blood to the top of the head and to ensure an adequate supply of blood for all organs at all times. But it must not be so high that blood vessels are damaged or burst, or that the heart has to work excessively hard in order to pump out blood against the pressure in the aorta.

As always when it is necessary to regulate something fairly precisely, the body has an effective system for regulating arterial pressure. This system, although complex in detail, is relatively simple in principle. As with all control systems, there are receptors for collecting information, there is a control centre which receives this information and decides what must be done and there are effectors which carry out the instructions of the control centre.

Pressure receptors or baroreceptors

The most important receptors which collect information about
arterial pressure are situated in the major arteries and in particular

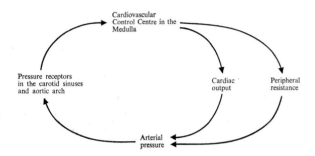

Fig.5.11. Outline of the control system which regulates arterial pressure.

in the arch of the aorta and the region known as the carotid sinus.
The carotid sinus is a dilatation where the common carotid artery
divides into internal and external branches. The receptors fire off
nerve impulses when the arterial wall is stretched and the greater
the degree of stretch the faster are the impulses generated. Since the
higher the pressure the more the vessel wall is stretched, the patterns
of impulses in the nerves from the receptors are a measure of the
arterial pressure. With each systolic pressure rise, the burst of
impulses gives the control centre an indication of the pressure level
in the major arteries.

The cardiovascular control centre

The main centre for the control of arterial pressure is in the medulla
oblongata at the lower end of the brain. Other parts of the brain
such as the hypothalamus have important parts to play but the
medulla seems to be the most important region. The centre receives
information from the pressure receptors about the situation in the
major arteries. If pressure is normal then the control mechanism
leaves well alone. If the pressure is too low the centre sends out
instructions to the effectors which tend to raise pressure, while if it
is too high the effectors are instructed to lower pressure.

Cardiovascular effectors

Pressure in the major arteries depends partly on how quickly blood is pumped into the aorta by the heart and partly on how quickly blood can leave the arteries via the arterioles. The faster the blood is pumped in, the higher will be the pressure: in other words the higher the cardiac output the higher the pressure will be. On the other hand, the more slowly the blood drains away via the arterioles the higher will be the pressure. If the arterioles offer a great deal of resistance to the flow of blood, the blood will drain slowly and pressure will tend to be high. If the arterioles are wide open, they will offer little resistance: blood will drain away rapidly and pressure will tend to be low. The resistance to flow offered by all the peripheral vessels and which depends mainly on the arterioles, is usually termed the peripheral resistance. The blood pressure therefore depends on the balance between cardiac output and peripheral resistance. If either the cardiac output or the peripheral resistance rise, pressure will tend to go up. If either falls, pressure will tend to go down. The control centre can therefore regulate arterial pressure by altering the cardiac output, the peripheral resistance or, more usually, both together. The main mechanisms available are as follows:

1. Cardiac output may be altered by changing

   a. The heart rate. Noradrenaline released by sympathetic nerves speeds the heart up, acetyl choline released by the vagus slows the heart down and adrenaline released into the blood by the adrenal medulla speeds it up.

   b. The vigour with which the heart contracts. The more vigorously the heart beats, the greater is the stroke volume (the amount of blood pumped out by the heart each beat.) The vigour of beating may be increased by noradrenaline released by sympathetic nerves and by adrenaline released by the adrenal medulla.

2. Peripheral resistance may be altered in many ways but probably most importantly by changing

   a. The activity of sympathetic nerves to the arterioles which release noradrenaline and which can cause constriction of almost all arterioles but especially those in the gut, skin and kidneys.

   b. The rate of release of adrenaline from the adrenal medulla. The adrenaline dilates arterioles in muscle and heart but constricts those elsewhere.

5

COMPLICATIONS OF PRESSURE REGULATION

The outline of pressure regulation just given is true of most circumstances, but there are a number of situations in which pressure in the major arteries may be normal, yet nevertheless the blood flow and oxygen supply to an organ may be defective. In these circumstances, pressure in the major arteries may be raised above normal in an attempt to restore to normal levels the blood and oxygen supply to a key organ. Three organs which seem to have extra defence mechanisms which attempt to safeguard their blood supply are the brain, the kidneys and the pregnant uterus.

The brain

If the drainage of cerebrospinal fluid is blocked in some way, the continued secretion of the fluid causes pressure inside the skull to rise. This rising pressure will tend to reduce the inflow of blood into the cranial cavity. Thus even though pressure in the carotid and vertebral arteries is normal, brain blood flow may be defective. The brain is clearly aware of this although as yet we do not understand the mechanisms involved. The result is that the control centre orders a rise in pressure in the major arteries in an effort to maintain a normal blood flow to the brain in the face of the increased resistance. Thus a rise in arterial pressure is an important clinical feature in patients whose intracranial pressure is rising.

Another factor altering blood pressure which is probably related to the need to supply adequate oxygen to the brain, is the oxygen level in arterial blood. If the arterial oxygen level falls (or if the carbon dioxide level or acidity rise) receptors in the aortic and carotid bodies (chemoreceptors) fire off impulses and blood pressure rises, presumably in an effort to increase the rate at which oxygen is supplied to the brain. The aortic and carotid bodies are tiny pieces of tissue close to the pressure receptors in the aortic arch and carotid sinus.

The kidneys

If the kidneys are to work effectively to remove waste material from the blood, they must receive a large supply of blood at an adequate pressure. If they do not receive such a blood supply, waste will accumulate in the body and eventually cause death. It is not uncommon for the kidneys to be damaged by disease or for the renal arteries to be partially blocked by atheroma or by an overgrowth of the tissue of the arterial wall. In either case the effect is that the kidney cannot carry out its functions satisfactorily. In an attempt to return renal function to normal, the kidney then seems to set in motion a train of events which raises the central arterial pressure to abnormally high levels. The details remain obscure but it is possible

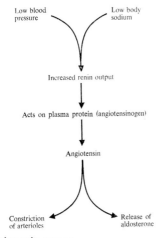

Fig.5.12. The renin-angiotensin system.

that the main events are as follows. Cells near to the glomeruli of the kidney (see chapter 7) release an enzyme known as renin. Renin can act on a protein in the plasma to break off from it a substance known as angiotensin which is a very powerful constrictor of arterioles. As well as constricting arterioles, angiotensin can act on the adrenal cortex to release aldosterone which increases the amount of salt and water retained in the body by the kidneys. Angiotensin and aldosterone appear to be responsible for the pressure rise.

The pregnant uterus

It is obvious that the pregnant uterus must have an excellent blood supply in order to allow the development of a healthy baby. If for some reason such as narrowed uterine arteries the blood flow to the uterus is impaired, there is some evidence that the uterus initiates a series of events which raises aortic pressure in a presumed attempt to raise uterine blood flow to normal. As yet the mechanisms involved are not understood.

RESPONSES OF THE CARDIOVASCULAR SYSTEM TO SPECIAL SITUATIONS

In this section the responses of the cardiovascular system as a whole to various special situations will be discussed.

Postural changes

Because veins are so thin-walled and stretchable, their degree of filling is very much affected by the force of gravity. This can readily be seen in a subject with prominent veins by asking him first to hold his hand above his head and then to lower it so that it hangs by his side. With the arm above the head the veins usually cannot be seen because the blood drains out of them under the influence of gravity. But with the hand by the side, gravity increases the pressure of blood in the veins and as a result they become prominent and full of blood. It someone is lying down flat the veins in the lower part of the body tend to be relatively empty of blood. On standing up gravity raises the pressure of blood in the leg veins which are therefore stretched and dilated. As a consequence of this, the filling of these dilated veins temporarily reduces the flow of blood back to the right heart. Since the veins when fully stretched can hold as much as 90 per cent of the total blood volume and since the heart can pump out only that blood which it receives, this pooling of blood in the veins will tend to lower the cardiac output and therefore also the blood pressure. If the blood pressure falls far enough, the blood supply to the brain will be impaired and the person will become unconscious. In normal individuals this sequence of events is prevented by a reflex which operates when a person moves from the lying to the upright position. Muscle, joint and inner ear receptors send information to the control centre that the person is standing up. Immediately the centre orders an increase in activity in the sympathetic nerves which go to the veins. This makes the muscle in the vein walls contract. The veins are thus stretched less than they would otherwise, be, the pooling of blood is limited and cardiac output and blood pressure are maintained. In people whose sympathetic system is defective because of disease, injury, surgical interference or drugs, the reflex is blocked and fainting is very likely to occur on suddenly standing up from a lying position. Fainting can happen in normal people who get out of a hot bath too suddenly as the warmth puts the vein walls into a very relaxed state.

Exercise

The cardiac output at rest is 4–5 litres/min and during exercise this may rise to 35 litres/min or even more. Despite this potential eightfold increase in cardiac output, arterial pressure rises by not more than 50 per cent and there must therefore be a considerable reduction in the peripheral resistance in order to accommodate the large cardiac output change. The dilatation of arterioles takes place in the skeletal muscles and heart. Arterioles in the gut and kidneys may constrict strongly. Thus blood is diverted from those organs which are of no immediate value in exercise to those which are vital.

Fainting

Fainting or syncope is a loss of consciousness due to a fall in pressure in the arteries supplying the brain. It may be initiated in two quite separate ways. First, any severe emotional shock can provoke a faint. Second, any persistent fall in cardiac output which tends to lead to a fall in blood pressure may lead to a faint. In both cases the effector mechanisms are the same: a great increase in vagal activity slows the heart and thus reduces cardiac output: simultaneously the blood vessels in the muscles dilate thus lowering the peripheral resistance. The net result is a sudden severe drop in blood pressure. This reduces the blood flow to the brain below a critical level and the person falls to the floor unconscious.

   Paradoxical though it may seem, a faint may be an important adaptive response which aims to maintain the cerebral blood flow in difficult circumstances. It may seem ludicrous that a tendency for arterial pressure to fall should be 'treated' by the control centre inducing a sudden further fall in pressure which leads to unconsciousness. Common causes of fainting are standing still in hot conditions for long periods (as with soldiers on parade or nurses watching a surgical operation) and loss of blood. When standing still in a hot place the leg veins become dilated. In the absence of leg movements, more than 80 per cent of the blood may become pooled in the veins in the lower part of the body. This so reduces the amount of blood effectively available to the heart that the cardiac output begins to fall and with it the blood pressure. If pressure cannot be maintained by vasoconstriction (most obviously noted by observing a dead white skin) then a faint is initiated. This rapidly forces the person to assume the horizontal position and so restores the flow of blood to the brain. A similar thing is true of haemorrhage: the horizontal position allows the heart to supply the brain most easily in conditions when the effective blood volume is reduced.

It follows from this that the worst thing anyone can do to someone who has fainted is to sit them up. The low blood pressure may then reduce the brain flow to dangerous levels and death has occurred when people have fainted in situations where they cannot fall such as a crowded train or a telephone booth. If you must do something for someone who has fainted, leave him flat and lift his legs into the air to help the drainage of blood back to the heart.

Haemorrhage

Bleeding or haemorrhage may be classified into three grades according to the nature of the pathophysiological response. In practice the three grades merge into one another with no sharp dividing lines.

A. Bleeding which is so slow that it causes no fall in either cardiac output or blood pressure. Examples are menstrual bleeding or bleeding from a chronic peptic ulcer. Extra water and salt are retained to compensate for the loss and the rates of synthesis of the plasma proteins and the formed elements are increased. Provided that nutrition and iron supplies are adequate, a healthy individual can easily compensate for this type of haemorrhage. The commonest cause of trouble is an inadequate intake of iron with consequent iron deficiency anaemia.

B. Bleeding which causes a fall in venous return and cardiac output but no fall in arterial pressure. This may occur if a small artery or vein is damaged. The blood volume, venous return and cardiac output fall and these changes tend to make blood pressure fall too. However the tendency for pressure to fall is detected by the pressure receptors and the control centre initiates constriction of arterioles in order to compensate for the falling cardiac output. Pressure is therefore maintained at normal levels: this can lull the doctor into a sense of false security because if he does not understand the physiological mechanisms, he may feel that because pressure is normal the patient is not bleeding.

The increase in peripheral resistance itself initiates changes which help to maintain blood volume. When an arteriole constricts the pressure in the capillary beyond it must fall. The osmotic pressure of the plasma proteins is unchanged and so the force drawing fluid into the capillary is greater than that pushing fluid out. There is therefore a tendency for fluid to move from the extravascular compartments into the blood. Plasma proteins and formed elements cannot be replaced in this way and so the blood becomes diluted with a fall in haemotocrit and haemoglobin levels.

If the haemorrhage is arrested by the haemostatic mechanisms (chapter 4), then the body compensates by more vigorous responses of the type outlined in A. If the haemorrhage is not halted the situation passes into stage C.

C. Bleeding which leads to a fall in venous return, in cardiac output and in arterial pressure. The cardiac output falls to levels so low that a normal blood pressure can no longer be maintained by increasing the peripheral resistance. Eventually a faint may be initiated and the pressure falls catastrophically. The main features of this type of haemorrhage are:

1. A falling blood pressure.

2. A weak pulse because the stroke volume is low.

3. A greyish-blue skin pallor. Vasoconstriction reduces the flow of blood and the slow flow allows haemoglobin to become completely deoxygenated.

4. Dry mouth and lax skin due to movement of fluid from the extravascular compartment into the blood.

5. Rapid, shallow breathing. The low rate of blood flow through the chemical receptors in the aortic and carotid bodies stimulates breathing (chapter 6).

6. Changes in the distribution of the cardiac output. Skin, gut and kidney blood flow are cut down drastically. In severe haemorrhage the lack of an adequate blood supply to the kidneys can cause renal damage and failure.

7. The outputs of ADH and aldosterone (chapter 7) are increased so that if the kidney is still working it holds back maximal amounts of salt and water.

Cardiovascular shock

Cardiovascular shock is said to occur whenever the cardiac output falls below the level required by the body. The signs and symptoms are similar to those of severe haemorrhage but they may be initiated in several different ways:

1. Cardiogenic shock. This occurs whenever the fall in cardiac output is primarily due to a defect in the heart such as a coronary thrombosis.

2. Shock due to a failure of venous return. There may be an actual loss of blood as occurs during haemorrhage or there may be a loss of fluid from the vascular system into the tissues because of damage to capillary walls as occurs in burns and crush injuries. Shock after surgery may be due partly to blood loss, partly to fluid loss into the tissues and partly to an inadequate fluid intake which prevents normal compensatory mechanisms from operating.

If blood has been lost, the only effective treatment is transfusion with whole blood. If compatible blood is not available, plasma or some plasma substitute should be used. Saline should be employed only in extreme emergency if nothing else is available because, since it contains no dissolved proteins or equivalent substances, most of it quickly leaves the blood and enters the extravascular tissues. With burns, since formed elements have not been lost to a great extent, plasma is the treatment of choice. In some cases in spite of all treatment the blood pressure and cardiac output fail to rise. This situation is called irreversible shock and the reason for it is unknown. It may be due to irreversible damage to the heart or to the arterioles.

6

Respiration

The respiratory system is a mechanism for moving oxygen from the air to the lungs and then into the blood and for moving carbon dioxide in the opposite direction. Because carbon dioxide when dissolved in water becomes an acid, the lungs are very important in the regulation of acid-base balance.

STRUCTURE

The exchange of gases between air and blood takes place in minute blind sacs known as alveoli. Each alveolus has a wall consisting of a single layer of flattened cells in intimate contact with blood capillaries. Here the air and the deoxygenated blood pumped into the lungs by the right side of the heart come into close contact. Since the amount of oxygen in the air is greater than that in the deoxygenated blood, oxygen automatically tends to flow down a concentration gradient from the air into the blood. The reverse happens with carbon dioxide. Thus, by passing through the lungs the venous-type blood

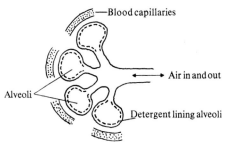

Fig.6.1. Outline of alveolar structure.

which is poor in oxygen and rich in carbon dioxide is converted to arterial-type blood rich in oxygen and relatively poor in carbon dioxide.

The air reaches the alveoli via a system of tubes consisting of trachea, bronchi and bronchioles. These contain smooth muscle fibres and the larger ones also contain cartilage for support. The smooth muscle in the bronchi and bronchioles is particularly interesting because its receptors are predominantly of the β type. This means that it is relaxed by adrenaline and by the β-stimulating drugs, thus explaining why these substances may be helpful during the respiratory distress associated with asthma.

All the tubes except those immediately preceding the alveoli which are known as alveolar ducts, are lined by an epithelium consisting of mucus-secreting goblet cells and ciliated cells. The cilia on the cell surfaces beat upwards towards the trachea and the throat thus generating a constant upward stream of mucus. This traps all types of foreign particles, including bacteria, and carries them upwards and outwards thus helping to keep the lungs clean. The cilia may be paralysed by toxic gases, by industrial fumes and by cigarette smoke, thus making it difficult to keep the lungs clean.

Only the alveoli themselves are concerned with gas exchange. The air in the nose, mouth, trachea, bronchi, bronchioles and alveolar ducts cannot make effective contact with the blood. Because it is not used in the actual process of gas exchange the space within the tubes leading from the nose and mouth to the alveoli is known as the 'dead space'.

THE MECHANISM OF BREATHING

The lungs are contained within the cavity of the chest. The lungs are covered by a smooth membrane known as the visceral pleura. The chest wall is lined by another smooth membrane known as the parietal pleura. Only the parietal pleura is pain-sensitive. The two layers of pleura are stuck together by a very thin layer of fluid, much as two microscope slides stick together when there is a thin film of water between them. The force involved is that of surface tension.

Lung tissue is highly elastic and outside the body the lungs shrink to a fraction of their volume in the chest. They are therefore kept expanded when in the body only by the force exerted by the thin film of pleural fluid which keeps the visceral and parietal pleura stuck together. If either the chest wall or an alveolus is punctured, so allowing air into the pleural cavity, the lung collapses giving the condition known as pneumothorax. Fortunately the two pleural

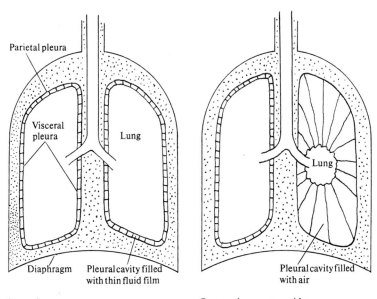

Fig.6.2. The lungs and pleural membranes showing how a pneumothorax can occur.

spaces are not continuous and unless both sides are damaged simultaneously only one side will collapse at a time.

The main muscles of respiration are the intercostal muscles between the ribs and the diaphragm. The diaphragm is the large sheet of muscle which separates the chest from the abdominal cavity. Breathing in is achieved by moving the ribs upwards and outwards and the diaphragm downwards so increasing the volume of the chest cavity. Because of the pleural mechanism the lungs must also expand and the pressure within them falls. Air then moves in to make the pressure inside the lungs equal to that in the atmosphere again.

Breathing out is achieved by the reverse process. The ribs move down and inwards and the diaphragm rises. This reduces the volume of the chest and the air within the lungs becomes slightly compressed.

This compression raises its pressure above atmospheric and the air moves out of the lungs until the pressure inside is again equal to that in the atmosphere.

During breathing in, the chest expansion pulls on the bronchi and bronchioles and opens them wider. During breathing out, the collapsing chest presses on the tubes and narrows them. This explains why in asthma where the tubes are narrowed by smooth muscle contraction, breathing out is often much more difficult than breathing in.

Coughing is a special pattern of breathing in and out which tends to expel foreign matter from the respiratory tubes. After an initial deep inspiration (breathing in), a forced expiration is made. During the expiration the glottis, the mechanism in the larynx which guards the entrance to the trachea, is initially closed so that no air can actually leave the chest. This means that pressure builds up rapidly and when the glottis suddenly opens, air rushes out at a speed which may approach 500 mph. This tends to carry solid and liquid matter up and out.

LUNG VOLUMES AND LUNG FUNCTION TESTS

Names for the various volumes of air within the respiratory system have now become widely accepted conventions. The tidal volume

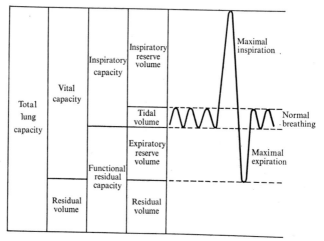

Fig.6.3. The relationships between the various volumes of air in the lungs.

is the volume of air breathed in and out during one respiratory cycle. The vital capacity is the volume of air moved out of the lungs when a maximal inspiration is followed by a maximal expiration. The residual volume is the amount of air left in the lungs after a maximal expiration. Some approximate normal values are shown in Table 6.1.

Table 6.1. Approximate values for the vital capacity and residual volume in various classes of people. Volumes are in litres.

	Young males	Young females	Old males
Vital capacity	4·8	3·2	3·6
Residual volume	1·2	1·0	2·4
Total lung volume	6·0	4·2	6·0

Many attempts have been made to develop reliable tests for measuring the state of lung function in patients, but most have proved either unreliable or suitable only for research purposes. Three may be used routinely:

1. *Vital capacity.* The patient is asked to take a deep breath in and then to breathe out again into an instrument which measures the volume and records it on a chart.

2. *Forced vital capacity (FVC) or forced expiratory volume (FEV).* In patients with narrowed bronchi and bronchioles the total vital capacity may be normal but the time taken to blow out the air may be greatly prolonged. In a normal individual about 80 per cent of the air is expelled in one second. The patient is therefore asked to take a deep breath in and then to breathe out as quickly as he can into a recording instrument. The volume of air breathed out in one second is recorded.

3. *Peak flow.* This is a rather simpler way of noting how quickly a patient can blow out air. He is asked to take a deep breath and then to blow out as quickly as possible into a device known as a peak flow meter which records the peak rate at which the air passes through it.

THE WORK OF BREATHING

The work which must be expended in order to breathe is used in overcoming two different types of resistance:

1. Friction. When air moves along the bronchi and bronchioles there is a frictional force between the moving air and the tube wall.

The faster the rate at which the air moves and the narrower the tube, the greater is the frictional resistance in relation to the volume of air which is moved.

2. Elasticity. The lungs and chest wall are both elastic. At the end of a quiet expiration the elastic forces balance out and no movement of the lungs and chest wall would occur if death suddenly occurred at this point. But if the lungs and chest are expanded or contracted beyond this point an elastic force must be overcome. As when stretching an elastic band, the effort required to move the chest increases the further one is from the equilibrium position. Thus when breathing is slow and deep, a great deal of effort is required to overcome the elastic forces.

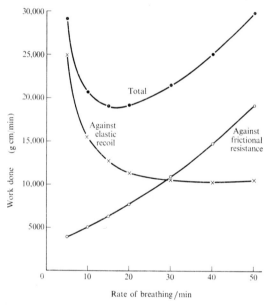

Fig.6.4. The relationship in breathing between the amount of work done in overcoming elasticity and the amount done in overcoming friction at various rates of breathing.

The frictional force which must be overcome is greatest when breathing is rapid and shallow while the elastic force is greatest when breathing is slow and deep. Obviously there must be some optimum intermediate rate of breathing when the sum of the two forces which must be overcome is at a minimum. In practice it has been found that the respiratory control centre is a remarkable computer which acts to minimize the amount of work which must be done during breathing. At any given ventilation rate (the ventilation rate is the respiratory equivalent of the cardiac output and is the volume of air moved in and out of the lungs in one minute), the brain adjusts the rate and depth of breathing so that the sum of the work done in overcoming friction and that done in overcoming elastic recoil is at a minimum. The control centre can perform this remarkable feat only because it receives a constant barrage of information from joint and muscle receptors in the chest wall and stretch receptors in the lung tubes.

Surface tension and the lungs

Some of the work done in overcoming the elastic recoil of the lungs is used to stretch the solid tissues, but some is used in stretching the thin layer of fluid which lines every alveolus. Inflating a lung is rather like inflating a million miniature soap bubbles. As almost anyone who has played with soap knows, when you blow a soap bubble you must keep blowing if the bubble is to continue expanding. If you stop blowing the bubble immediately starts to collapse. This is because of the force of surface tension. Molecules in a thin liquid film resist being pulled apart: when an active force pulling them apart ceases they rush together again.

The force of surface tension may be greatly reduced by chemicals known as detergents which reduce the attraction of water molecules for one another. In the presence of a detergent the effort which must be expended in order to pull the molecules apart is much less. It is therefore not surprising that the body has evolved a mechanism whereby detergent is secreted into the alveoli. This reduces the surface tension of the thin fluid film to about one tenth of what it would otherwise be and greatly reduces the work of breathing.

The effectiveness of the detergent (often known as 'lung surfactant') is best seen by noting what happens when the detergent is absent. This occurs in some babies who are born prematurely. They are unable to manufacture the surfactant and they develop a condition known as respiratory distress syndrome, in which it is obvious that the baby is having to work incredibly hard in order to breathe. This is not surprising because in the absence of surfactant it is necessary to work about ten times as hard as normal in order to overcome the surface tension.

CONTROL OF VENTILATION RATE

The ventilation rate can be defined as the volume of air moved in and out of the lungs every minute. The ventilation rate which is required depends to a large extent on the amount of muscular exercise being performed, although of course even in the resting state some oxygen is required and some carbon dioxide is produced. But during exercise much more oxygen is used up and much more carbon dioxide is produced, so that if normal blood levels of these gases are to be maintained the ventilation rate must increase accordingly.

How does the body know what the ventilation rate should be? There is a typical control system with sensory receptors, a control centre and effectors. The control centre is in the lower part of the brain known as the medulla and it is usually called the respiratory centre. The effectors are the muscles of the chest wall, mainly supplied by the thoracic spinal nerves, and the diaphragm, supplied by the

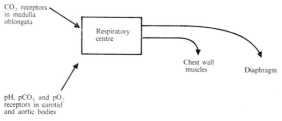

Fig.6.5. The respiratory control system.

phrenic nerve which leaves the spinal cord in the neck and travels down through the thorax. The receptors are in several different places. The most important ones monitor the chemical composition of arterial blood. Normally the partial pressure of oxygen (pO_2) is 95–100 mm Hg, that of carbon dioxide (pCO_2) is about 40 mm Hg and the pH is about 7·4.

The receptors

The most important ones are as follows:

1. Receptors in the brain near the respiratory centre. These are well placed to monitor the arterial blood passing through the brain and also possibly the cerebrospinal fluid. They are sensitive to carbon

dioxide. A rise in pCO_2 stimulates ventilation while a fall in pCO_2 reduces ventilation. The brain receptors are not sensitive to oxygen lack in that oxygen lack does not stimulate ventilation by acting on them. A deficiency of oxygen at the brain level in fact depresses ventilation because it interferes with the functioning of nerve cells in the respiratory centre.

2. Receptors in the carotid body and the aortic body. These are small pieces of tissue near the carotid sinus and in the wall of the arch of the aorta: they lie close to the corresponding pressure receptors. They are sensitive to three separate chemical stimuli, the pH and the levels of oxygen and carbon dioxide in arterial blood. A rise in acidity, a fall in pO_2 and a rise in pCO_2, all stimulate the receptors and lead to a rise in ventilation rate. The reverse changes lower the ventilation rate. By acting on these receptors (sometimes known as the peripheral chemoreceptors) oxygen lack therefore stimulates breathing: this is in contrast to its action on the brain.

3. Receptors in the joints which signal when joint movements occur. These warn the respiratory centre that exercise is beginning and are responsible for an initial increase in ventilation which occurs in anticipation of the later changes in carbon dioxide and oxygen levels.

The respiratory control centre

The information from all the receptors is sent to the respiratory centre which can thus build up a clear picture of what is happening. If carbon dioxide is accumulating in arterial blood, this means that the lungs are not working rapidly enough to get rid of all the carbon dioxide that is being produced in the tissues. If oxygen levels are low in the arteries, this means that oxygen is being used up more rapidly than it is being supplied by the lungs. If acids other than carbon dioxide are accumulating in arterial blood, this means that something is wrong in the tissues: abnormal amounts of acid may be produced because of oxygen lack or insulin lack or acids may not be being excreted normally because of kidney failure.

The respiratory centre continually adjusts the ventilation rate in order to maintain the composition of the arterial blood normal and constant. Under most circumstances it seems to be most sensitive to changes in pCO_2, probably because quite small changes in the level of carbon dioxide can seriously upset acid-base balance. Only when oxygen lack is severe or when abnormal acids are present in high concentration do these stimuli become more important than the carbon dioxide level.

Once the respiratory centre has decided what ventilation rate is required, it then has to estimate what combination of rate and depth of breathing will achieve this with the minimum of expenditure and effort. In order to do this, it relies on information from muscle and joint receptors in the chest wall and from receptors in the lungs. The end result is usually very appropriate as outlined in the previous section.

THE TRANSPORT OF OXYGEN

Oxygen is not very soluble in water. At the normal pO_2 in the lung alveoli and in arterial blood (about 100 mm Hg) only about 3 ml of dissolved oxygen can be carried by each litre of blood. This is clearly insufficient to supply the needs of the body, for even at rest an adult uses about 250 ml of oxygen per minute. The problem is solved because the red cells contain a red pigment known as haemoglobin. This has the remarkable property of easily and reversibly combining with oxygen, one molecule of haemoglobin (Hb) picking up four molecules of oxygen. When the haemoglobin concentration of the blood is normal (around 140–150 g/litre) and when each Hb molecule is carrying four molecules of oxygen, the red cells in one litre of blood carry about 200 ml of oxygen, over sixty times the amount which can be carried in dissolved form.

Haemoglobin which is fully oxygenated is bright red, while Hb without oxygen is purplish in colour. When a patient appears bluish because his blood vessels are filled with deoxygenated blood, he is said to be cyanosed. There are two main forms of cyanosis:

1. *Peripheral cyanosis*. When the rate of blood flow to the skin is reduced because of cold or haemorrhage, the blood that remains in the skin may become deoxygenated and blue because it is stagnant. However, in these circumstances the blood in the central arteries is usually normally oxygenated as can be seen by looking at the tongue. The small blood vessels of the warm tongue are always wide open and so the colour of the tongue reflects the colour of arterial blood.

2. *Central cyanosis*. With this condition both the tongue and the skin are blue because the cyanosis is due to inadequate oxygenation of arterial blood and indicates serious failure of either lung function or heart function.

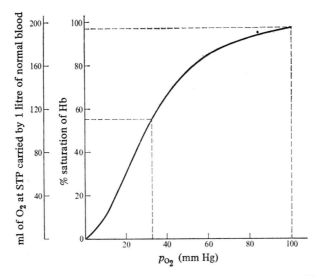

Fig.6.6. The relationship between the pO_2, the percentage saturation of haemoglobin and the amount of oxygen carried by a litre of normal blood.

Haemoglobin dissociation curve

The relationship between the pO_2 of the blood and the amount of oxygen carried by Hb is an unusual one. It can be described by the dissociation curve shown in Fig.6.6. At very low partial pressures below about 20 mm Hg, Hb does not attract oxygen very strongly and little oxygen combines with it. But between 20 and 60 mm Hg, Hb attracts oxygen very strongly indeed and the amount of oxygen bound to it rises very rapidly. At 60 mm Hg the Hb is carrying about 75–80 per cent of all the oxygen it is capable of transporting. Above this point, as the pO_2 rises, the amount of oxygen carried by Hb rises relatively slowly again. By the time a pO_2 of 100 mm Hg is reached the Hb is more than 95 per cent saturated. The importance of the shape of the curve lies in the following points:

1. At normal ventilation rates, with a normal alveolar pO_2 of about 100 mm Hg, the Hb is almost completely saturated and each litre of normal blood carries about 200 ml of oxygen. Since the resting cardiac output is about 5 litres/min, the total amount of oxygen pumped out by the heart at rest, is around 1 litre/min. Since the resting oxygen consumption is about 250 ml/min there is an ample safety margin.

2. The upper end of the curve is flat. This means that arterial pO_2 must fall below 60 mm Hg before the transport of oxygen is seriously impaired. Even at this partial pressure each litre of normal blood carries 160 ml of oxygen and 800 ml of oxygen per minute are transported around the body, so that the supply is still ample at rest.

3. Below a pO_2 of 60 mm Hg the curve is steep and Hb gives up its oxygen readily and rapidly. This means that the oxygen is made available to the tissues while the pO_2 is still relatively high.

The importance of the last point is clearly seen in carbon monoxide poisoning. Carbon monoxide is an extremely toxic substance found in coal gas and vehicle exhaust fumes. Natural gas usually contains little or none of it. Carbon monoxide is so toxic because it combines with Hb much more readily even than oxygen does and it therefore prevents the oxygen becoming attached. However carbon monoxide can kill even when only 25 per cent of the Hb combining points are

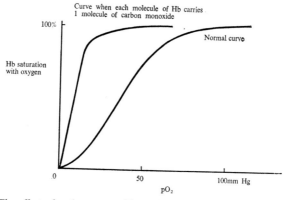

Fig.6.7. The effect of carbon monoxide on the relationship between oxygen and haemoglobin.

occupied by it, leaving 75 per cent still carrying oxygen. One might have thought that this would have left an ample safety margin, but the real trouble arises because the carbon monoxide alters the shape of the dissociation curve. When carbon monoxide has combined with one of the four slots on an Hb molecule, the other three take up oxygen much more readily than usual and even at a pO_2 of only 20 mm Hg the Hb may be 80 per cent saturated. Looking at it the other way, the new shape of the curve means that the Hb will cling on to most of its oxygen until the blood pO_2 has fallen to 10–15 mm Hg. At this blood pO_2 brain cells will be dead. Therefore, even though there may be plenty of oxygen in the blood it is useless because it cannot be given up and supplied to the tissues at a high enough pO_2.

Hyperbaric oxygen

This term literally means oxygen at high pressure. If a patient is put into a special chamber where he can breathe pure oxygen at three atmospheres pressure, the partial pressure in the lungs and arterial blood can be raised to about 2200 mm Hg. At this pO_2 between 60 and 70 ml of oxygen can be carried in simple dissolved form by each litre of blood, so by-passing the need for haemoglobin. The main uses of hyperbaric oxygen are:

1. Carbon monoxide poisoning. The high pressure oxygen avoids the need for Hb transport and also tends to displace the carbon monoxide from its combination with Hb.

2. Respiratory distress syndrome in infants.

3. After coronary thrombosis when the damaged heart cannot pump blood effectively through the lungs, it cannot itself receive an adequate supply of blood and thus enters a vicious circle which can end only in death. It has been claimed that high pressure oxygen can improve the outlook although this has been disputed.

4. In the treatment of infections with bacteria which are killed by oxygen.

5. During the treatment of cancer by X-rays. It has been found that well-oxygenated tumours are more susceptible to the action of X-rays and that the results of treatment are improved if he is exposed to high pressure oxygen while the cancer is being irradiated.

TRANSPORT OF CARBON DIOXIDE

When carbon dioxide enters the capillary blood from the tissues, small amounts stay in the plasma either in dissolved form or in combination with plasma proteins, but most of it passes straight into the red cells. The red cells are therefore almost as important in the transport of carbon dioxide as they are in the transport of oxygen. In the red cells two main things may happen to the carbon dioxide:

1. It may combine with Hb to form a substance known as carbamino-Hb. About 25 per cent of the carbon dioxide which enters the blood in the capillaries is carried to the lungs in this form.

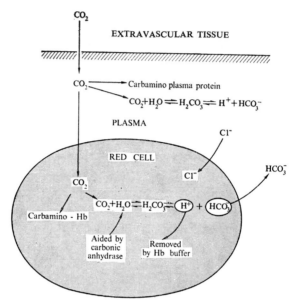

Fig.6.8. The disposal of the carbon dioxide which enters the blood in the capillaries.

2. It may react with water to give carbonic acid and the carbonic acid may then split up to give H^+ and HCO_3^- ions.

$$CO_2 + H_2O \rightleftharpoons H_2CO_3 \rightleftharpoons H^+ + HCO_3^-$$

In the red cells there is an enzyme known as carbonic anhydrase which speeds up by about 5000 times the combination of carbon dioxide and water. The carbonic acid breaks down to give hydrogen and bicarbonate ions because these two ions are continually being removed from the red cell. This is because Hb is a very effective buffer and combines with and neutralizes many of the H^+ ions, as follows:

$$Hb^- + H^+ \rightleftharpoons Hb . H$$

One positive and one negative charge disappear so that the red cell remains neutral. However as the reaction moves to the right, the concentration of bicarbonate builds up rapidly and soon rises well above the bicarbonate concentration in the plasma. Because of this concentration gradient bicarbonate diffuses out of the red cell into the plasma. The loss of negative ions leaves the inside of the red cell relatively positive and so chloride ions diffuse in from the plasma in compensation. This is sometimes known as the chloride shift (Fig. 6.8.). All these changes are reversed when the blood gets to the lungs and the carbon dioxide diffuses out of the red cells into the alveoli where the pCO_2 is relatively very low. About 75 per cent of the carbon dioxide which enters the tissue capillaries is carried to the lungs in the form of bicarbonate.

The red cells therefore play a potentially important role in acid-base balance and this is discussed further in chapter 11.

THE PULMONARY CIRCULATION

The pulmonary circuit from the right ventricle to the left atrium is much smaller than the systemic circuit of the circulation from left ventricle to right atrium. The pressures required are much less than those in the systemic circuit and pulmonary artery pressures are in the region of 8–15 mm Hg as compared with 70–120 mm Hg in the normal aorta. An important consequence of this is that capillary blood pressure in the lungs is very low. In fact it is much lower than the plasma protein osmotic pressure and so the force drawing fluid out of the alveoli into the blood is much greater than the force pushing fluid in the opposite direction. Thus the alveoli tend to be kept fairly dry and are lined by only a very thin layer of fluid which is probably actively secreted in order to keep the cells in good condition. Because the alveoli are kept relatively dry, the barrier to oxygen flow from air to blood and to carbon dioxide flow in the reverse direction is kept to a minimum.

If for any reason (such as a coronary thrombosis) the left ventricle fails, blood may pile up in the lung capillaries. Its pressure may rise above the plasma protein osmotic pressure and fluid may move out into the alveoli giving the condition known as pulmonary oedema. In the mildest form, the 'wet' lung seriously interferes with gas exchange. In the severe form the alveoli, bronchi and bronchioles may quickly be filled up with pink frothy fluid which comes up the trachea and out of the nostrils. Unless quickly treated, the acute form of severe pulmonary oedema soon ends in death.

7

The kidneys
and urinary tract

The main functions of the kidneys are the regulation
of the amount of water and dissolved ions in the body, the excretion
of waste matter and the manufacture of erythropoietin, the hormone
which regulates red cell synthesis (chapter 4).

OUTLINE OF STRUCTURE

The principal features of kidney structure can be seen in a longitudinal
section through the organ. There is a dark outer cortex with a paler
inner medulla. In the centre there is a cavity, the renal pelvis, into
which the urine drains. The urine is carried from the pelvis to the
bladder by the ureters.

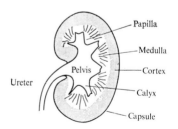

Fig.7.1. Section through a kidney showing the main regions.

The basic units out of which the kidneys are constructed are the
nephrons. Each human kidney has about a million of them. Each
nephron is a blind-ended tube made of a single layer of cells. It
follows a tortuous route from the cortex where the first process of

urine formation takes place, to the medulla where the urine finally enters the pelvis. The blind end of each nephron is a cup-like

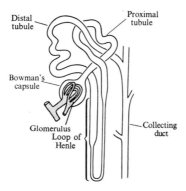

Fig.7.2. A nephron.

structure known as Bowman's capsule. From this cup there leads a highly convoluted tube known as the proximal tubule which is still within the cortex. The tubule then takes a surprising course, dipping right down into the medulla and coming back again in a U-shaped structure known as the loop of Henle. There then follows another tortuous section known as the distal tubule. Finally the distal tubules join together to form collecting ducts which run down through the medulla to drain into the renal pelvis.

The details of kidney blood supply are very important. The arteries divide to give arterioles which enter the cup of the Bowman's capsule (afferent arterioles). In the capsule they break up into a mass of capillaries known as the glomerulus. The capillaries then join up to form a second arteriole (efferent arteriole) which leaves the capsule. Associated with the afferent arteriole are a group of cells known as the juxta-glomerular apparatus which make the enzyme renin.

Once the efferent arterioles leave the glomeruli they do not send the blood into veins on its way to the heart. This is why they are called arterioles rather than venules. Instead they break up into a second set of capillaries which supply the proximal and distal tubules, the loops of Henle and the collecting ducts. This second set of capillaries then join up to form venules and veins.

The kidney has a rich sympathetic nerve supply. The fibres go to two main parts of the organ.

1. The arterioles, especially the afferent arterioles. These sympathetic fibres which release noradrenaline are important in adjusting renal blood flow and especially in reducing blood flow during exercise and haemorrhage when the blood is diverted to other organs.

2. The juxta-glomerular apparatus where the sympathetic impulses can alter the amount of renin produced.

GLOMERULAR FILTRATION

Urine is initially formed in the glomeruli and Bowman's capsules. Because the renal arteries and afferent arterioles are short and relatively wide, pressure in the glomerular capillaries is considerably higher than pressure in any other capillaries in the body, being 60–70 mm Hg instead of the usual 20–30 mm Hg. This means that the capillary blood pressure is considerably higher than the osmotic pressure of the plasma proteins. There is therefore a tendency for all substances which can pass through the glomerular capillary wall to do so rapidly. This means that all the blood constituents apart from the plasma proteins, the platelets and the red and white cells pass into the Bowman's capsule. The important things to note about the normal glomerular filtrate, as it is called, are the following:

1. The formed elements of the blood are absent. Red and white cells do not normally appear in urine.

2. Protein is absent and therefore protein in the urine is always an indication of some abnormality.

3. Apart from the absence of protein, platelets and red and white cells, the chemical composition of the filtrate is identical to that of the plasma.

The blood flow to both human kidneys is in the region of 1200 ml/min in the resting state and the plasma flow is therefore about 700 ml/min. About one fifth of the plasma is filtered off in the glomeruli and so the glomerular filtration rate, the amount of fluid filtered per minute, is in the region of 120–140 ml/min in a normal adult. This means that each day 150–180 *litres* of fluid enter the nephrons. The normal daily urine output is less than 2 litres and so 99 per cent of the fluid which enters the nephrons must be salvaged and returned to the blood.

THE PROXIMAL TUBULE

The greater part of the salvage operation takes place in the proximal tubule. The most important substances which are reabsorbed from the tubular fluid and returned to the blood are the following:

1. Sodium. There is an active pumping mechanism which removes sodium ions from the tubules and transfers them to the blood.

2. Chloride. When each positive sodium ion is reabsorbed, an excess of negative charge is left in the urine while there is a relative excess of positive charge in the tubular cells. Since like charges repel while unlike charges attract, the electrical balance is kept partly because chloride ions follow the sodium.

3. Bicarbonate ions are reabsorbed by a complex mechanism which is partly dependent on hydrogen ion secretion into the urine and on sodium reabsorption.

4. Potassium is actively reabsorbed.

5. Glucose is actively reabsorbed by a special pumping mechanism. Normally all the glucose is removed from the tubular fluid by the end of the proximal tubule and none appears in the final urine. However, the pumping mechanism has a limited capacity and if too much glucose is delivered to it, it cannot cope and some of the glucose passes straight through and out into the urine. This does not normally occur until the concentration of glucose in the plasma (and in the glomerular filtrate for the two have the same composition) rises above about 180 mg/100 ml.

6. The reabsorption of water depends on two main factors:

a. The protein osmotic pressure of the blood in the capillaries which supply the proximal tubule. This is raised above normal because in the glomeruli about one fifth of the plasma is lost from the blood but none of the protein is lost. The protein concentration is therefore increased, so raising the osmotic pressure and the force drawing fluid from the proximal tubule.

b. The continual removal of sodium, chloride, bicarbonate, glucose and other dissolved materials from the tubular fluid means that there is a tendency for their concentrations to be slightly higher in the blood than in the tubular fluid. In order to maintain the balance, because of osmotic forces water follows the dissolved material. This second factor is probably considerably more important than the protein osmotic pressure in water reabsorption.

All the glucose, all the potassium and most of the bicarbonate is normally removed from the tubular fluid by the end of the proximal tubule. About 80–90 per cent of the water and sodium are also removed leaving relatively small quantities to be dealt with by the rest of the nephron.

THE LOOP OF HENLE

The functions of the loop of Henle are understood in broad outline but the details remain obscure The loop operates what is known as a 'counter-current multiplying system' in such a way that the medulla becomes loaded with sodium and its accompanying negative ions. In the kidney cortex the total concentration of ions in the interstitial fluid, in the plasma and in the cells is similar to that in any other tissue in the body. But in the deepest part of the medulla the total ionic concentration may be 3–4 times higher than normal. The ionic concentration of the interstitial fluid, of the cells and of the plasma rises steadily from the outer cortex to the inner medulla and this rise is brought about by the operation of the loop of Henle. The mechanism of the rise will not be discussed here but its importance will be seen in the next sections.

DISTAL TUBULE AND COLLECTING DUCT

As far as dissolved substances are concerned, the main thing which happens in the distal tubule is the reabsorption from the urine of sodium, in exchange for the secretion into the urine of hydrogen and potassium ions. Either hydrogen or potassium can be excreted in

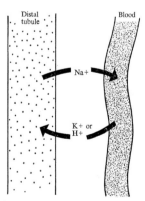

Fig.7.3 . Ionic movements in the distal tubule.

exchange for sodium: this means that if the hydrogen ion secretion rate falls the potassium secretion rate must rise and vice versa. Some of the consequences which may occur as a result of this mechanism are:

1. If the blood becomes alkaline, few hydrogen ions are secreted by the distal tubule. This may lead to the loss of considerable quantities of potassium instead.

2. If the blood becomes acid, many hydrogen ions are secreted. Potassium then tends to be retained in the body.

3. If the body is severely depleted of potassium ions, hydrogen ions must be excreted by the kidneys in exchange for sodium. This hydrogen ion secretion occurs even in the presence of alkaline blood, leading to the paradoxical situation of an alkaline blood and an acid urine.

The distal tubule and collecting duct are very important in the regulation of water excretion. Their role in this will be fully discussed in the section of hormonal control of the kidney.

ACID EXCRETION

Hydrogen ions are secreted into the urine by both the proximal and the distal tubules. More are secreted by animals on a meat diet than by those on a vegetarian diet. The lowest pH which the urine can reach is about 4·5. In order to buffer the hydrogen ions which are secreted into the urine three separate mechanisms are available:

$$1. \quad H^+ + HCO_3^- \rightleftharpoons H_2CO_3 \rightleftharpoons H_2O + CO_2$$
$$2. \quad H^+ + HPO_4^= \rightleftharpoons H_2PO_4^-$$
$$3. \quad H^+ + NH_3 \rightleftharpoons NH_4^-$$

Fig.7.4. The buffering of hydrogen ions in the urine.

1. The hydrogen ions may combine with bicarbonate to give carbonic acid, the latter then splitting up to give water and carbon dioxide. The carbon dioxide diffuses back from the urine into the blood and is excreted by the lungs.

2. The hydrogen ions may combine with phosphate. Most of the phosphate in plasma and in the glomerular filtrate is in the form of HPO_4^{--} ions. Each one of these can combine with and remove from solution one hydrogen ion to give $H_2PO_4^-$.

3. The hydrogen ions may combine with ammonia. The distal tubular cells contain large amounts of an amino acid known as glutamine. When large amounts of hydrogen ions are being secreted, glutamine can split up to give glutamic acid and ammonia. The ammonia enters the tubular fluid where it combines with hydrogen ions to give ammonium ions (NH_4^+).

HORMONAL CONTROL OF THE KIDNEY

Two hormones, vasopressin or anti-diuretic hormone (ADH) and aldosterone are established as important controllers of renal function. Recent work suggests that other hormones such as growth hormone and prolactin may also be important.

Anti-diuretic hormone

This is secreted by the posterior lobe of the pituitary gland. The posterior pituitary is quite different from the anterior pituitary in that it has a very rich nerve supply. The nerve cells have their cell bodies in the part of the brain known as the hypothalamus and their axons travel down the pituitary stalk to the posterior pituitary. ADH is actually manufactured by the nerve cells in the hypothalamus and then passes down the axons to the posterior pituitary where it is released when nerve impulses pass along these fibres. The action of ADH is on the distal tubule and collecting ducts. In its absence,

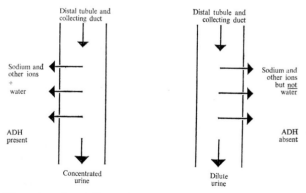

Fig.7.5. The action of anti-diuretic hormone.

as far as water is concerned, these structures behave like steel tubes: they will not allow water to pass from the tubular fluid into the blood. The fluid which reaches the distal tubules from the loop of Henle is fractionally less concentrated than plasma as far as ions are concerned. In the absence of ADH, when sodium and other substances are reabsorbed in the distal tubules water cannot follow and so must pass on to the urine. As the solids are removed, the urine therefore becomex more and more dilute. There is a disease known as diabetes insipidus, the Latin name literally indicating the production of large amounts of tasteless urine. This disease occurs when little or no ADH is produced because of some malfunction of the pituitary or hypothalamus. As much as 10–20 litres of very dilute urine may be poured out every day. The patient must of course drink enormous quantities in order to maintain the water content of his body.

In contrast, when ADH is present in large quantities, the distal tubules and collecting ducts are completely permeable to water. This means first, that when any solid material is reabsorbed from the urine into the blood, an equivalent amount of water follows thus ensuring that the urine does not become more dilute than the plasma. Second, as the urine passes in the distal tubules and collecting ducts down through the medulla, it travels through regions where the interstitial fluid and cells have a steadily increasing concentration, which in the inner parts of the medulla may be 3–4 times higher than the ionic concentration of the plasma. The concentration of the fluid outside the ducts is therefore greater than that inside and if the duct walls are permeable to water, water will move out of the ducts in order to maintain osmotic equilibrium. The net result is that in the presence of ADH the urine comes into equilibrium with the interstitial fluid through which it is passing and eventually becomes 3–4 times more concentrated than the plasma. By adjusting the concentration of ADH in the blood, the permeability of the distal tubules and collecting ducts can be adjusted to any desired level between complete permeability to water and complete impermeability. Thus urine of the desired concentration can be produced.

Several different factors govern the output of ADH:

1. The osmotic pressure of the blood passing through the hypothalamus where there are receptors for monitoring it. If the blood becomes more dilute its osmotic pressure falls: this suggests that there is too much water in the body and the output of ADH is

reduced. If the blood becomes more concentrated, its osmotic pressure rises and ADH output is increased in order to keep water in the body.

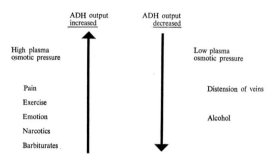

Fig.7.6. Factors influencing ADH output.

2. The degree of distension of the great veins. Stretch receptors in the thin-walled veins give a rough indication as to whether the circulatory system is over-filled with blood. If it is over-filled, ADH output is reduced in order to allow fluid to escape from the body.

3. Pain, exercise and emotion all increase ADH output, possibly because in these situations the rapid accumulation of fluid in the bladder is inconvenient.

4. Some drugs, notably alcohol, suppress ADH output and cause a diuresis (an increase in urine flow).

5. Other drugs, notably narcotics and barbiturates, increase ADH output and reduce urine volume.

Aldosterone

Aldosterone is a steroid hormone manufactured by the outermost layer of the adrenal cortex. Its action is on the distal tubule where it increases the reabsorption of sodium and therefore, in the presence of ADH, of water as well. As the sodium is reabsorbed, potassium and hydrogen ions tend to be excreted in exchange. The factors which govern the amount of aldosterone secreted are not yet fully clear and are the subject of much research. The present position is outlined in Fig.7.7.

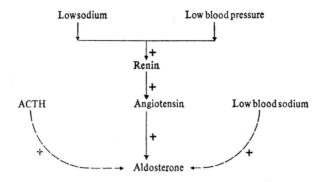

Fig.7.7. Possible factors influencing aldosterone output.

Prolactin and growth hormone

It has recently been demonstrated that both prolactin and growth-hormone can act on the kidneys to reduce the excretion of water, sodium and potassium. This action has been little investigated as yet, but it may be important during the menstrual cycle and during pregnancy and lactation.

INDICATORS OF RENAL FUNCTION

It is helpful to have some relatively simple indicators of the extent of renal damage in patients with kidney disease. The simplest thing of all is to look at the urine and to check it for the presence of red cells and protein. Both are normally absent and either if present indicates some form of renal damage.

Another useful test is the estimation of the blood urea concentration. Urea is the end product of the breakdown of the nitrogen-containing parts of amino acids. It is formed from ammonia by the liver and excreted almost exclusively in the urine. It is freely filtered at the glomeruli and is not actively reabsorbed: some urea is passively reabsorbed along with the water, but large amounts are excreted. If the glomerular filtration rate falls, the rate of excretion of urea also falls and the blood urea concentration rises. However there is a wide safety margin and the blood urea concentration does not rise sharply until the glomerular filtration rate has fallen to well under half its normal level. As the amount of renal damage increases beyond this point however, the blood urea level rises rapidly.

A somewhat more precise indication of the amount of renal damage that has occurred may be obtained by the use of the concept of clearance. We know that the concentration of a freely filtered substance is exactly the same in both the glomerular filtrate and the plasma. Suppose there were a substance which, once it had been filtered, was neither reabsorbed nor secreted during passage of the urine along the rest of the nephron. If this happened then all the substance filtered would appear in the urine. By collecting the urine over a period of time and analysing it, it would therefore be possible to know how much of the substance had been filtered by the glomeruli during that period. Since the concentration of the substance would

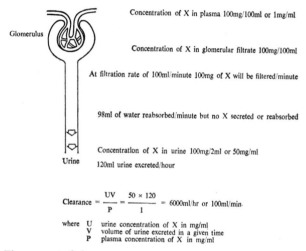

Fig.7.8. The concept of clearance.

be the same in both plasma and glomerular filtrate, it would be possible by taking a blood sample to know the concentration of the substance in the glomerular filtrate. Now the total amount of substance X filtered in a given time must be equal to the concentration of X in the glomerular filtrate multiplied by the volume of the filtrate in that time.

i.e.

Amount of X filtered = concentration of filtrate × volume of filtrate.

By analysing the urine and measuring its volume we can know the total amount filtered, by analysing the blood sample we know the concentration in the glomerular filtrate and it is therefore possible to calculate the volume of fluid filtered during a given time. The glomerular filtration rate gives a rough indication of how many glomeruli are functioning normally.

A number of substances are used for these 'clearance' studies as they are called. One which is natural in the body is creatinine, a breakdown product of the substance creatine which is found in muscles. The concentration of creatinine in the plasma is remarkably steady in any one individual and it is not reabsorbed at all by the nephron. It is secreted to a small extent and this means that more creatinine appears in the urine than was filtered at the glomeruli. In consequence, if creatinine is used for a clearance study the glomerular filtration rate is overestimated a little. However, because the creatinine clearance test is so easy to perform it is used frequently. A 12 or 24 hour collection of urine is made and the total amount of creatinine in it is estimated. During this period a blood sample is taken in order to estimate the concentration of creatinine in the plasma and in the glomerular filtrate and the filtration rate is estimated.

There are a number of other substances, such as inulin (a carbohydrate), which are not normally found in the body but which when infused into the blood are freely filtered at the glomeruli and are neither reabsorbed nor secreted. These substances can therefore be used to estimate glomerular filtration rate relatively accurately. However they must be steadily infused during the test and this makes them more difficult to use than creatinine.

MICTURITION

Urine is conveyed from the renal pelvis to the bladder by the ureter. The ureters are muscular tubes which contract rhythmically in waves so forcing the urine along. Where each ureter reaches the bladder there is a valve mechanism which allows urine to enter the bladder but not to pass in the reverse direction. This is important because it means that infection of the bladder (cystitis) cannot normally be transmitted backwards up to the kidneys. This is not true in pregnancy: for unknown reasons, but possibly because of the presence of high levels of progesterone, the smooth muscle of the ureters and the valves is in a very relaxed state. This means that especially during contraction of the bladder, the urine can pass backwards up towards the kidneys.

The wall of the bladder is made up primarily of criss-crossing smooth muscle fibres. These fibres of the wall (the detrusor muscle) are relaxed except when micturition is actually taking place. Another smooth muscle, the internal sphincter, guards the exit from the bladder. It is aided by a skeletal-type striated muscle, the external sphincter. Both sphincters are normally tightly contracted to prevent the escape of urine.

In the wall of the bladder there are stretch receptors which send information about the degree of fullness of the bladder to a control centre in the lowest part of the spinal cord. When filling reaches a critical level, the control centre, using both sympathetic and parasympathetic effector nerves, reverses the resting pattern of bladder muscle activity. The sphincters relax and the detrusor contracts, forcing out the urine. In paraplegic patients and in babies the reflex

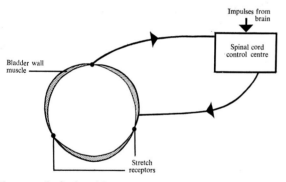

Fig.7.9. The control of micturition.

is not under conscious control and occurs automatically. In normal children and in adults the reflex can be blocked or activated by nerve impulses descending the spinal cord from the brain. These impulses may act on the control centre and may also alter the state of bladder receptors. If the smooth muscle adjacent to the receptors contracts, they fire off impulses just as they do when they are stretched by filling of the bladder. Relaxation of the smooth muscle reduces the impulse activity. Thus the brain can control micturition by modifying the activity both of the receptors in the bladder which supply the information and also of the control centre itself.

8

The alimentary tract

The main function of the alimentary tract is the transfer of food materials from the outside world to the blood. In the process, three separate stages are involved:

1. The food must be moved along the gut.

2. The food must be broken down into small molecules (digested).

3. The food must be transferred across the gut wall into the body (absorbed).

OUTLINE OF STRUCTURE

The gut throughout its length consists of inner mucosal and outer muscular layers. The function of the mucosal layer is to produce secretions which lubricate and digest the food and to absorb the

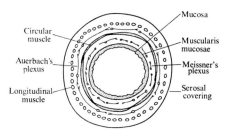

Fig.8.1. The layers of the gut wall.

digested material. The function of the muscular layer is to propel the food along. The mucosa and the muscular layer are separated by an extremely thin layer of smooth muscle known as the muscularis mucosae. Outside this are much thicker inner circular and outer longitudinal layers of muscle. Complex nerve plexuses, usually known as Meissner's and Auerbach's, lie between the muscle layers.

Nerve supply

Three main types of nerve fibre supply the gut:

1. Sensory nerves, which carry information about stretch of the gut wall and about the pH and chemical composition of the gut contents.

2. Parasympathetic nerves, which are responsible for stimulating the gut movements which propel the food along. The vagus supplies the gut up to the middle of the large bowel. The last part of the large bowel is supplied by parasympathetic nerves from the sacral region of the spinal cord.

3. Sympathetic nerves, whose primary importance is in the control of the blood supply. They may also stimulate the action of the smooth muscle sphincters which guard the exits from and entrances to each section of gut.

The plexuses of nerves within the gut wall can do a remarkable amount by themselves and even when all the external nerves are cut can still to some extent coordinate the movement of food.

Smooth muscle

The gut smooth muscle contracts spontaneously but the spontaneous activity can be modified by nerve activity and by circulating adrenaline. Acetyl choline released from parasympathetic nerves increases the activity of the main muscle in the gut wall and relaxes the sphincters. Adrenaline (epinephrine) relaxes the main gut muscle and stimulates the sphincters to contract, so stopping the movement of food. The part played by the sympathetic nerves is uncertain, but they may stimulate the sphincters to contract.

The movements of gut smooth muscle are of two main types:

1. *Churning movements* (*segmentation*), in which the muscle contracts and relaxes mixing the gut contents but not pushing the food along very much.

2. *Propulsive movements* (*peristalsis*), in which a coordinated wave of relaxation followed by contraction passes along the intestine. Peristalsis may be initiated by stretch of the gut wall by a ball of

food. There is then reflex relaxation in front of the ball and reflex contraction behind it, so pushing the food along.

THE MOUTH AND OESOPHAGUS

In the mouth the food is chewed to break it up into small pieces and to lubricate it by mixing it with saliva. The saliva also dissolves some of the food so allowing it to be tasted. Saliva contains an enzyme, amylase, which can begin the conversion of starch to the disaccharide, maltose. However this digestive function is probably not very significant: its main purpose is probably to clear the mouth of fragments of food. Cessation of salivary secretion leads to foul breath within an hour and dental decay within a week. Saliva is an alkaline, watery fluid, rich in sodium, potassium, chloride and bicarbonate. It also contains mucus which acts as a lubricant. The mucus and the watery secretion are produced by different cells. There are four main types of salivary gland:

1. *Tiny groups of cells* on the surfaces of the mouth and pharynx which secrete a mucus-rich fluid.

2. *The sublingual gland* beneath the tongue contains mainly mucus-secreting cells.

3. *The parotid gland* on the side of the face in front of the ear, contains cells which secrete a watery, enzyme-rich fluid.

4. *The submandibular glands* tucked underneath the jaw contain both types of cells.

Secretion of mucus is brought about mainly by sympathetic nerves, while parasympathetic impulses cause a profuse flow of watery saliva. Several different sorts of sensory stimulus may lead to activation of these nerves and salivary gland secretion. The main ones are:

1. Smelling or anticipating food as shown by Pavlov's dogs (chapter 3).

2. The act of chewing.

3. Chemical stimulation of taste receptors by food in the mouth. Bitter substances are by far the most effective.

Swallowing

Swallowing may be initiated either voluntarily or reflexly by touching certain areas near the back of the mouth. Anyone who has sat in a dentist's chair knows the power of the reflex and the difficulty of controlling it once initiated. The control centre for the reflex is in the lowest part of the brain, the medulla oblongata.

Swallowing begins with the tongue pressing up against the hard palate (the roof of the mouth) and pushing a ball of food back in to the pharynx at the back of the mouth. Once the food is in the pharynx all voluntary control of the reflex is lost. Muscles in front of the food relax while those behind it contract. The wave of relaxation and contraction pushes the food down into the stomach. The movement of both food and fluids depends on muscular activity rather than on gravity and it is possible to hang upside down and to swallow effectively.

The entry to the stomach is guarded partly by muscle in the wall of the oesophagus and partly by the action of the diaphragm which nips the oesophagus. These mechanisms normally prevent the stomach contents moving backwards up the oesophagus. If because of some abnormality or some temporary malfunction the acid stomach contents do pass up into the oesophagus, the acid stimulates pain receptors giving the familiar sensation sometimes known as 'heartburn'.

THE STOMACH

An outline of structure is shown in Fig.8.2. The stomach is a large muscular bag which has the following functions:

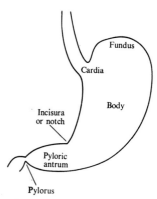

Fig.8.2. Outline of stomach structure.

1. To store food and pass it on to the intestines in a controlled, steady manner.

2. To begin the digestion of proteins.

3. To mix up and soften the food by its regular churning movements.

4. To secrete 'intrinsic factor' which is essential if vitamin B_{12} is to be absorbed. The intrinsic factor is a mucoprotein which combines with the vitamin. The combination, but not the vitamin alone, can then be bound to the wall of the intestine and the vitamin taken into the body.

5. To absorb a few substances. In general the stomach is not a major organ of absorption, but some substances such as alcohol and aspirin are relatively rapidly absorbed by it.

Stomach movements

Spontaneous waves of activity begin near the top of the stomach where the oesophagus enters and moves regularly down to the pylorus about three times per minute. Hormones and nerve activity do not alter the rhythm but they do alter the intensity of the contractions. Acetyl choline released by the vagus fibres to the stomach is by far the most important factor in maintaining normal gastric movements. Section of the vagus as part of the surgical treatment of peptic ulcer severely interferes with the normal emptying of the stomach: it must be combined with a so-called 'drainage' operation. In such an operation the exit of food from the stomach is made easier either by widening the pylorus (pyloroplasty) or by making an additional exit directly from the bottom of the stomach to the small intestine (gastro-enterostomy).

When the stomach has recently been emptied of food, the contractions are very feeble. As hunger develops, they increase in intensity but then become very weak again when the stomach is filled: gradually they become stronger and each one then forces a spurt of food into the duodenum.

Several mechanisms, all starting with the activation of sensory receptors in the duodenum, are important in modifying the rate of stomach emptying. Chyme (the mixture of food from the stomach) in the duodenum, slows down the rate at which food enters the duodenum particularly if the chyme is acid or fatty. Three mechanisms are involved:

1. The receptors initiate impulses which cause the release of a hormone from the duodenal wall. This is known as enterogastrone and it circulates in the blood and reduces stomach activity.

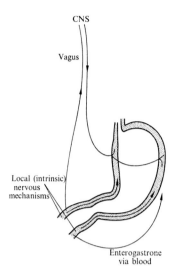

Fig.8.3. The control of stomach movements by the entry of food into the duodenum.

2. The receptors initiate impulses which travel to the stomach through the nerve plexuses in the gut wall and inhibit stomach smooth muscle contraction.

3. The receptors send information to the central nervous system which then reduces the activity of the vagus nerve, again diminishing the intensity of stomach contractions.

Gastric secretion

The main part of the stomach surface is lined by simple cells which secrete mucus and a small amount of an alkaline fluid which helps to protect the stomach from the action of its own gastric juice. Leading down from the surface are many deep pits, the gastric glands, which contain the cells which secrete the gastric juice. There are three main types of cells:

1. Those near the neck of the gland secrete mucus which spreads over the surface of the stomach as a protective layer, trapping the alkaline fluid and preventing acid and enzymes getting at the stomach surface cells.

2. Deeper in the gland are chief cells which produce an inactive enzyme precursor known as pepsinogen.

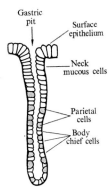

Fig.8.4. An outline of gastric gland structure.

3. Also deep in the gland are the parietal or oxyntic cells which secrete hydrochloric acid and possibly intrinsic factor.

The glands in the cardiac area where the oesophagus enters the stomach contain mucus-secreting cells only. Those in the pyloric area near the exit contain mucus-secreting and enzyme-secreting but no acid-secreting cells. Those in the main body of the stomach contain all three cell types.

Pepsinogen is secreted in an inactive form because if it were made in active form it would break up the proteins in the secreting cells themselves. It is activated by conversion to pepsin on contact with acid: the acid splits off a small part of the pepsinogen molecule so exposing the active part of the enzyme. Once some pepsin has been formed, the pepsin itself can then convert pepsinogen to pepsin. The pH of the normal stomach contents is 2–3 because this is the optimum pH for the protein-splitting activity of pepsin. Little if any digestion of carbohydrates or fats takes place in the stomach.

STIMULI TO SECRETION. The secretion of gastric juice is conventionally divided into three phases which merge into one another.

1. *Cephalic phase.* This refers to the gastric secretion which can be brought about when no food has yet entered the stomach. On smelling, seeing or thinking of food, and especially on putting food into the mouth, there is an outpouring of gastric juice. The information from the receptors is carried to the control centre in the medulla oblongata in the lower part of the brain. This activates the vagus which releases acetyl choline and which stimulates the gastric glands

to secrete. This phase is known as the cephalic phase because it depends on the control centre in the brain.

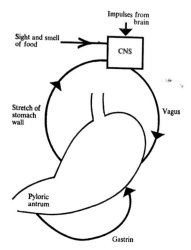

Fig.8.5. The control of gastric secretion.

2. *Gastric phase.* This refers to the secretion which occurs in response to the actual entry of food into the stomach. Chemical and stretch receptors in the stomach wall, particularly in the pyloric region, lead by three mechanisms to an increase in the flow of gastric juice.

   a. By the intervention of the nerve plexuses in the stomach wall.

   b. By sending impulse to the control centre in the CNS which then increases the activity of the vagus.

   c. By causing the release of a hormone called gastrin from the region of the stomach known as the pyloric antrum. Gastrin enters the venous blood, is carried to the heart and pumped out by the arteries again to the stomach. On reaching the gastric glands it powerfully stimulates their secretion.

3. *Intestinal phase.* If in an experiment, food is placed directly into the small intestine without first passing through the stomach, gastric secretion is stimulated. Thus the digestion of food in the stomach is promoted by the presence of food in the intestines. The mechanisms are not known.

THE PANCREAS

The pancreas is the single most important source of digestive juices. Its secretion contains enzymes which can split up all three of the major foodstuffs, fat, carbohydrate and protein. The enzymes all work best at a pH which is slightly on the alkaline side of neutral. They will not work at the acid pH of gastric juice and so it is important that the gastric secretions should be neutralized. This is achieved partly by the bile but mainly by the large amounts of bicarbonate present in the pancreatic secretions.

The pancreas is, of course, also an important endocrine gland because it contains the islets of Langerhans which secrete insulin and glucagon.

The cells which secrete the digestive juices are arranged in groups called acini which empty into tiny tubules. These join up until eventually they form the main pancreatic duct which empties into the duodenum. It often shares a common emptying point with the bile duct. There is a powerful muscle (the sphincter of Oddi) which controls the emptying of bile and pancreatic juice into the duodenum.

The vagus nerve and the hormone gastrin can both stimulate pancreatic secretion but they are probably much less important than two other hormones, secretin and pancreozymin. Secretin causes a copious flow of watery juice, while pancreozymin stimulates the secretion of an enzyme-rich juice. Normally the two act together. They are both manufactured in the wall of the duodenum and are both released into the blood when food enters the duodenum from the stomach. The hormones are then carried by the blood around to the pancreas. Acid is a potent stimulator of the flow of secretin while partially digested foods, especially proteins and fats, stimulate the flow of pancreozymin.

THE BILE

Bile has two main functions. It acts as an excretory channel for certain substances, notably cholesterol and the breakdown product of haemoglobin, bilirubin, and it also contains the bile acids which are important in the digestion of fat. This section is concerned with the control of bile secretion.

Bile is manufactured in the liver and between meals it is stored in the gall bladder. In the gall bladder, sodium, chloride, bicarbonate and water are all absorbed from the bile into the blood. Cholesterol, bilirubin and the bile salts are all left behind and because of the absorption of water they may become 5–10 times more concentrated than in the bile freshly secreted by the liver. Partly as a result of this concentration, some of the solid material (especially cholesterol and to a lesser extent bilirubin and other substances formed from it, which are collectively known as the bile pigments) tends to precipitate out giving gall stones which may sometimes escape from the gall bladder and block the bile ducts. However concentration cannot be the only factor in the formation of gall stones since it occurs in everyone, while gall stones, although common, are by no means universal.

Control of the flow of bile into the duodenum depends on two factors; control of the rate of bile secretion by the liver and control of the emptying of the gall bladder. The main factors which alter the rate of bile secretion are probably the following:

1. Activity of the vagus nerve.

2. The hormone secretin, released by the duodenum when food enters the duodenum from the stomach.

3. The presence of bile salts in the blood carried to the liver by the portal vein.

About half an hour after feeding, the gall bladder contracts and pours its bile into the duodenum just as food is beginning to enter the small intestine from the stomach. This contraction depends on two mechanisms:

1. Food in the duodenum stimulates sensory receptors which then lead to reflex activity in the vagus. The vagal fibres to the gall bladder release acetyl choline which causes muscle contraction.

2. Food in the duodenum causes release of a hormone called cholecystokinin from the duodenal wall. Cholecystokinin circulates in the blood and causes strong contractions of the gall bladder. It is possible that cholecystokinin may be the same substance as secretin or even pancreozymin.

THE SMALL INTESTINE

The small intestine consists of the short duodenum leading on to the much longer jejunum and ileum. It secretes a digestive juice, sometimes known as the succus entericus, whose composition has not yet been precisely defined. The major functions of the small intestine are to provide a site where digestion can occur and to absorb the digested food. The biochemistry of digestion and absorption is dealt with in 'Essential Biochemistry, Endocrinology and Nutrition'.

In order to carry out its functions, the small intestine must be able to churn the food up and move it along and must be able to provide good conditions for absorption. The movements are similar to those which occur in the rest of the gut and they have been described at the beginning of the chapter.

Absorption

Absorption of the digested food into the body must take place through the gut wall. Since the greater the surface area of the gut wall the more rapidly absorption can take place, it is not surprising that the surface area of gut available is increased in three different ways:

1. The whole mucosal surface is thrown into folds.

2. The mucosal folds are covered by minute finger-like projections known as villi: each villus has a rich blood supply and also a large central lymphatic known as a lacteal. Most of the digested food passes into the blood, but the fats tend to enter the lacteals.

3. Each cell surface facing the gut is itself covered with myriads of almost unbelievably tiny projections known as microvilli. These greatly increase the surface area available.

In the cells which line the gut there are active mechanisms for moving many substances into the body. Those which are actively shifted in this way include sodium, glucose and amino acids. The movement of these solids tends to leave the gut contents of a lower osmotic pressure than the plasma and so water automatically follows them into the blood. Some other absorptive mechanisms which are not infrequently affected in disease are:

1. Calcium. The absorption of calcium depends on gastric acidity and on the availability of adequate supplies of vitamin D. The way in which the acid operates is unknown but it may help to shift the calcium into a more soluble form. Patients who have defective acid secretion, either naturally or after surgery for peptic ulcer, tend to become calcium deficient. If there is too much phosphate in the food the calcium may be precipitated in a very insoluble form and which cannot be absorbed. This sometimes occurs in new born infants fed cows' milk, which has a much higher phosphate content than human milk.

2. Iron. The normal absorption of iron, again for uncertain reasons, requires the secretion of normal amounts of gastric acid. Iron deficiency anaemia is common in those whose acid secretion is defective.

3. Fat soluble vitamins (A, D, E and K). The absorption of these depends on the normal absorption of fat. If anything interferes with fat absorption (e.g. inadequate bile or pancreatic juice secretion), then vitamin deficiencies may follow.

4. Vitamin B_{12}. As mentioned at the beginning of the chapter, the absorption of vitamin B_{12} depends on the secretion of a mucoprotein 'intrinsic factor' by the stomach. The intrinsic factor combines with the vitamin. The complex is then bound by the wall of the ileum and the vitamin is absorbed. In the absence of intrinsic factor the disease known as pernicious anaemia develops.

Absorption of all valuable solid materials is complete by the time the end of the ileum is reached. There is a valve which guards the exit from the ileum to the large intestine and which normally prevents reflux of the contents of the large intestine into the small intestine. This is important because the contents of the small intestine are normally sterile and creamy-white in colour. Bacterial infection of the small intestine may lead to serious problems of absorption. The small intestine normally delivers 400–600 ml of material to the large intestine every day. Most of this consists of water, indigestible material and remnants of dead cells which are continually being shed from the gut surface.

LARGE INTESTINE

The large intestine has three main functions:

1. It offers a place for the storage of unwanted material until it can be excreted as faeces at a convenient time.

2. It absorbs water so that the fluid material which leaves the small intestine (chyle) is reduced to about 25 per cent of its volume by the time it is excreted as faeces.

3. It offers a home to a large colony of bacteria. It is being increasingly recognized that these bacteria synthesize vitamins and may be important sources of vitamins of the B group, especially folic acid.

The large intestine consists of a blind sac, the caecum with its attached appendix, the long ascending, transverse and descending colons and the rectum where the faeces is finally stored.

Defaecation

Defaecation is stimulated by the stretching of receptors in the wall of the rectum. This stretching may arise from two sources:

1. Distension of the rectum with faeces.

2. Contraction of the muscle of the rectal wall. The receptors behave as though they are fixed between the ends of the muscle fibres and so when the muscle fibres contract the receptors between them are stretched. The rectal wall muscle may be stimulated by voluntary action or, as in diarrhoea, by the presence of abnormal bacteria or toxins.

In infants or in older people who have lost control of defaecation because of damage to the spinal cord, distension of the rectum to a certain critical level automatically fires off the defaecation reflex. There is a control centre in the lower part of the spinal cord which orders the following effector acts when the sensory input to it reaches trigger point:

1. Peristalsis occurs in the large intestine forcing faeces along to the rectum.

2. The muscles in the rectum contract, the circular ones raising pressure and the longitudinal ones pulling the rectum up and over the faeces it contains.

3. The internal (smooth muscle) and external (striated muscle) sphincters relax and the faeces is automatically expelled.

In normal individuals the reflex may be voluntarily suppressed by impulses coming down the spinal cord from the brain to the control centre and also by the relaxation of the rectal muscle which takes the tension off the receptors. On the other hand, when the time is appropriate, the reflex may be voluntarily encouraged by instructions sent to the control centre and by contraction of the rectal muscle which stimulates the receptors. The expulsion of faeces may also be voluntarily assisted by raising the intra-abdominal pressure by means of the Valsalva manoeuvre. This familiar act consists of closing the glottis, pulling the diaphragm down, and contracting the muscles of the abdominal wall. The complete voluntary control of defaecation depends on an intact spinal cord and on intact somatic and parasympathetic peripheral nerves.

A great deal of nonsense is talked about the need to empty the bowels once per day. It is true that this is the most usual pattern, but there is immense individual variation: some entirely normal individuals may empty their large intestines once a week and others three times a day. Neither pattern need be abnormal provided that it is the usual one for that individual. A *change* in bowel habit, however, is a very important clinical feature as not infrequently it indicates disease.

The discomfort which is associated with constipation is primarily due to stretching of the large intestine and has little if anything to do with the absorption of toxins. The sensation may be rapidly produced by placing a balloon in the rectum and blowing it up and may be instantly relieved by letting down the balloon.

CLINICAL ASPECTS OF GUT FUNCTION

Most disorders of gut function can be more easily understood if the physiology is known. Three of the more important aspects of disordered physiology will be discussed here.

Fluid losses

Fluid losses from the gut are not uncommon. Vomiting leads to a loss of gastric secretion, while diarrhoea may lead to loss of the contents of the large intestine. Patients with an ileostomy may lose fluids from the small intestine (an ileostomy is a way of by-passing the large intestine if the latter is severely diseased or has to be surgically removed: the end of the ileum is brought out through the anterior abdominal wall and empties into a bag). Excess fluid loss from any part of the gut leads to the loss of water, of sodium and accompanying negative ions, and of potassium. In some ways the potassium loss is the most important, partly because it tends to be forgotten, partly because the amount of potassium in the extra-cellular fluid is relatively small and partly because even small variations in plasma potassium concentration may have serious effects on heart function. It is very important to ensure that any fluid and ions which are lost are promptly replaced.

The effect of the fluid loss on acid-base balance depends on which fluid is lost. Usually fluid lost from the stomach is acid and so an excess of alkali is left behind (metabolic alkalosis). Fluid lost from below the duodenal level is usually alkaline and so leaves an excess of acid behind in the body (metabolic acidosis).

Peptic ulcers

An ulcer occurs when epithelial tissue is lost from any surface in the body leaving a raw area. A peptic ulcer is an ulcer which occurs in a part of the gut exposed to 'peptic' (gastric acid-containing) juice; in effect this usually means ulcers in the stomach and duodenum.

An ulcer could occur either because of a lack of the normal factors which protect the gut surface or because of an excess of the powerful destructive components of gastric juice. Mucus is probably the most important protective agent while acid and pepsin are the destructive ones. There is a lack of agreement among research workers as to what is most important, but tests of acid secretion have yielded interesting results. Acid secretion may be tested by putting a tube into the stomach of a resting person who has not eaten for 12 hours or more. The contents are sucked out and then suction is continued for an hour in order to estimate the so-called basal rate of acid secretion. An injection of histamine (preceded by an anti-histamine to avoid unpleasant side effects) or of a synthetic relative of gastrin known as 'pentagastrin' is then given. Both these substances are very powerful stimulators of acid secretion. The acid is then collected for another hour giving an estimate of the maximal rate of secretion. These tests have now been carried out in very large numbers of patients and it has been found that duodenal ulcer patients tend to have high acid secretion rates, while gastric ulcer patients tend to have low acid secretion rates. This suggests that duodenal ulcers may be due to an excessive secretion of gastric juice while gastric ulcers may be due to defective defence mechanisms. The idea that gastric ulcer is associated with defects in the stomach wall is supported by the fact that gastric ulcers are associated with gastric cancer and with pernicious anaemia due to lack of secretion of intrinsic factor. Duodenal ulcers are not associated with either cancer or pernicious anaemia.

Malabsorption

Malabsorption, as the word implies, is a condition in which the food passing through the gut is not absorbed normally. Large amounts pass straight through the small intestine into the large bowel and out in the faeces, causing diarrhoea and malnutrition. The condition has two fundamental causes:

1. A failure of digestion. If food is not digested it cannot be absorbed even though the absorptive mechanisms of the small intestine are working normally. Since the most important of all the digestive juices comes from the pancreas, pancreatic disease frequently causes malabsorption. Lack of normal bile secretion causes a failure of fat absorption. There are also a number of diseases in which enzymes important in digestion are congenitally absent. These are most important in infancy and are discussed in 'Essential Biochemistry, Endocrinology and Nutrition'.

2. A failure in the absorptive process itself because of damage to the wall of the small intestine. The most important causes of this are coeliac disease and sprue. Coeliac disease is in part a failure of digestion because the gut seems incapable of digesting fully the protein, gluten, which is found in wheat. Some of the products of partial digestion are toxic and damage the wall of the small intestine causing atrophy of the villi and failure of absorption. A complete cure can be achieved by withdrawing wheat products from the diet. In sprue, the wall of the small intestine degenerates in much the same way as in coeliac disease but the cause seems to be quite different although it is by no means fully understood. One possibility is that a change in the types of bacteria present in the gut means that they consume folic acid instead of producing it. Sprue can usually be relieved by giving large doses of folic acid and by altering the gut bacteria again by the use of antibiotics.

9

Reproduction

Human reproduction, as everyone knows, is of the sexual variety. The process begins with the formation of eggs (ova) in the female ovaries and of spermatozoa (sperm) in the male testes. In the act of sexual intercourse, if it occurs at the right time, the two are brought together and the fertilized egg or zygote results. This becomes implanted in the uterus which has been prepared for its reception and develops over approximately 280 days in normal circumstances to a fully formed infant. In the process of labour (parturition), the infant is pushed into the outside world and the cycle normally ends with the feeding of the infant with milk from the mother's breasts.

MALE REPRODUCTIVE FUNCTION

The primary reproductive organs in the male are the testes. These

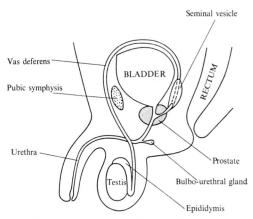

Fig.9.1. Outline of the structure of the male genital tract.

are responsible for the production of both sperm and of male sex
hormones (androgens) of which testosterone seems to be the most
important. For normal function the testis is dependent upon the
hypothalamus and pituitary. The rest of the male internal and
external genitalia shown in outline in Fig.9.1. essentially consist of
mechanisms for delivering the sperm to the female in a healthy
condition.

Control by pituitary and hypothalamus

Before puberty the testes are small and produce only minute amounts
of testosterone. The testosterone circulates in the blood and its
presence is detected by the part of the brain known as the hypothalamus. The hypothalamus is connected by means of the special
system of blood vessels known as the pituitary portal system to the
anterior pituitary. The anterior pituitary produces two hormones,
the so-called gonadotrophic hormones, which can affect the testes.

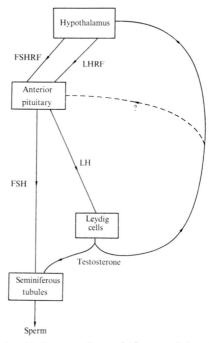

Fig.9.2. The relationship between the seminiferous tubules of the testis which
produce sperm, the Leydig cells which produce testosterone, the hypothalamus
and the anterior pituitary.

These are follicle-stimulating hormone (FSH) and luteinizing hormone (LH): they were originally named because of their effects in the female, but since it is now known that the male and female pituitary hormones are identical it has become conventional to call the two hormones FSH and LH whether one is discussing males or females. LH in the male is still sometimes known as interstitial cell stimulating hormone or ICSH.

Before puberty FSH and LH are secreted by the anterior pituitary in negligible quantities. This is because they depend for their secretion on two substances released from the hypothalamus into the pituitary portal system. These two are FSH-releasing factor and LH-releasing factor. Before puberty, the releasing factors are secreted by the hypothalamus in only very small amounts: the minute quantities of testosterone produced by the testes seems able to prevent the hypothalamus from secreting larger amounts of the releasing factors.

Puberty and the functions of the testes

At puberty something which is not yet understood happens to the hypothalamus. It becomes much less sensitive to the testosterone in the blood and the minute quantities of androgen can no longer prevent the hypothalamus from secreting large amounts of the releasing factors. And so, in turn, the pituitary begins to secrete large amounts of FSH and LH. These two hormones circulate in the blood and act on the testes to convert them to the adult form.

The testes contain three main types of cell:

1. *Germ cells* involved in the production of vast numbers of sperm. During the cell divisions which occur, the number of chromosomes is reduced from the 46 found in all other cells in the body to the 23 found in a sperm. A similar process occurs during egg formation so that when a sperm containing 23 chromosomes fuses with an ovum containing 23 chromosomes the result is a zygote with the normal number of 46 chromosomes. A mature sperm is a remarkable cell consisting primarily of a huge head which carries the nucleus with its chromosomes, a middle piece containing many mitochondria whose function is to supply energy and a long tail which utilizes this energy to lash the fluid in which the sperm is bathed, so enabling it to swim.

2. *Sertoli cells* of uncertain function but which may supply nutrients for the sperm.

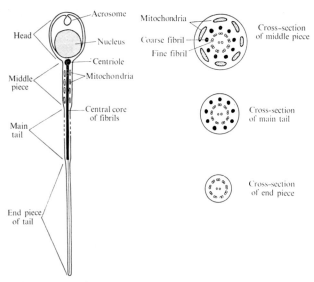

Fig.9.3. The structure of a sperm.

3. *Interstitial cells* (Leydig cells) which manufacture testosterone.

Broadly speaking, LH stimulates the secretion of testosterone and the testosterone acts with FSH to promote the development of mature sperm. FSH and LH together therefore stimulate the testis to grow and to change its function to the adult type. The hypothalamus still remains dependent on testosterone for controlling the amounts of releasing factors which it secretes, but very much larger amounts of testosterone are now required. However, if testosterone concentration in the blood becomes too high, FSH and LH secretion rates are reduced until testosterone concentration falls back to the desired level. If it becomes too low, FSH and LH output are increased in order to return testosterone levels back to normal.

Secondary sexual characters

At puberty the increased output of testosterone causes the familiar changes which convert a boy into a man. The main ones are:

1. The internal and external genitalia and in particular the penis grow to adult size.

2. Because of changes in the vocal chords, the voice breaks and becomes deep.

3. The skin becomes coarser and much more grease is secreted.

4. The muscles develop and strengthen and the personality tends to become more aggressive.

5. Pubic and axillary hair grow. The male pattern of pubic hair has a point going up towards the umbilicus while the female pattern is a flat-topped triangle.

6. The hair line over the temples recedes to give the adult male pattern.

7. The fusion of the growing points of the bones (the epiphyses) is accelerated, so tending to terminate growth.

THE FEMALE SEXUAL CYCLE

Female sexual function is much more complex and much less well understood than sexual function in the male. The primary organs are the ovaries which have two main functions, the production of ova and the manufacture of hormones.

The formation of ova

At birth the ovary contains between 200,000 and 500,000 structures known as primordial follicles, each of which can give rise to a single mature egg. More than half of these degenerate during childhood but the 100,000 plus which are left at puberty are more than enough to supply one egg per lunar month for the 30–40 years of female reproductive life.

Before puberty no mature ova are released because the amounts of FSH and LH released by the pituitary are too small; the secretion of the hormones seems to be suppressed by tiny amounts of oestrogen (female hormone) from the ovaries acting on the hypothalamus. At puberty, as in the male, the output of FSH and LH rises, the ovary develops and fully formed eggs begin to be released at monthly intervals.

In an adult, at about the time of menstrual bleeding, several primordial follicles enlarge and the cells surrounding them (the membrana granulosa cells) multiply. Within a few days, for unknown reasons and by unknown mechanisms just one of these primordial follicles is selected: it enlarges rapidly while the others which had been enlarging degenerate. A fluid filled cavity soon appears within the granulosa cells giving a structure known as a Graafian follicle.

The cells surrounding the follicle, the theca interna and externa, secrete female hormones. The Graafian follicle grows and moves towards the surface of the ovary. Eventually, usually about 12–14 days after the beginning of the previous menstrual period, the

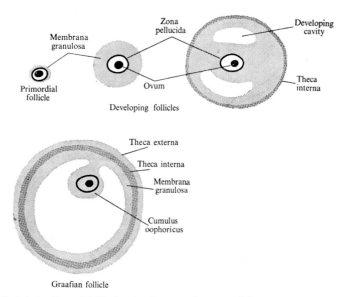

Fig.9.4. Outline of follicular development (not to scale).

follicle ruptures, releasing the ovum into the abdominal cavity, normally close to the opening of the Fallopian tube. The egg is then carried by the movements of the tube and of the cilia which line its walls, down to the uterus.

The follicular cells which remain in the ovary after the egg has been released are rapidly vascularized by the growth of new blood vessels. Under the stimulus of the increased blood supply the cells grow rapidly. Many of them become yellow in colour and because of this the ruptured follicle becomes known as the corpus luteum. The corpus luteum is an active secretor of female hormones and remains functional until about the time of the next menstrual flow when it degenerates.

The female hormones

As in the male, the primary sex organ, the ovary, secretes only very small amounts of hormone before puberty. After puberty, mainly under the influence of LH, the ovaries secrete much larger amounts of hormones which fall into two groups known as the oestrogens and the progestins. Oestradiol is probably the most important natural oestrogen and progesterone the most important natural progestin, but there are many other substances in each group, both natural and synthetic.

The oestrogens are primarily responsible for the changes which occur at puberty. The main changes are:

1. Development of the internal and external genitalia.

2. Growth of the breasts and rounding of the body contours due to selective deposition of fat.

3. Changes in psychological make-up.

4. The beginning of menstruation (menarche).

5. Growth of pubic and axillary hair. Adrenal androgens may be more important than ovarian hormones in this, since hair growth is normal at puberty even when the ovaries are congenitally absent (Turner's syndrome).

Progesterone is the hormone which is secreted by the corpus luteum and its actions are discussed in the next sections.

The hypothalamus, pituitary and ovaries

The control of hormone secretion is much more complex in the female than in the male and is relatively poorly understood. During the first half of the menstrual cycle until just before the egg is released (ovulation), the rate of oestrogen secretion rises steadily but little if any progesterone is produced. A few hours before ovulation actually occurs, there is a sharp rise in the output of progesterone. During the second half of the cycle (luteal phase) both oestrogens and progesterone are present in relatively high concentrations but their levels fall again as the corpus luteum degenerates and menstrual flow begins. No one doubts that this pattern is dependent on pituitary hormones but most of the details remain obscure. The one outstanding feature is that there is a very sharp peak in the output of LH just around the time of ovulation. This peak in LH secretion almost certainly stimulates the release of progesterone and of the egg. In most women the peak and the subsequent ovulation occur at about the mid-point (12th–16th days after menstrual flow starts) of a normal four-week cycle. In women with irregular cycles ovulation usually occurs about 14 days *before* the following menstrual flow.

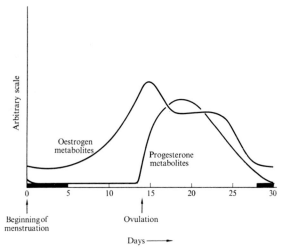

Fig.9.5. The urinary excretion of metabolites of oestrogen and progesterone during the menstrual cycle.

It seems to be the first part of the cycle which is irregular while the second almost invariably lasts for two weeks.

Some animals, notably the rabbit, do not have a cycle as such. The ovary is ready to release eggs at almost any time. When copulation takes place, the nervous stimuli associated with it cause a burst of LH release from the pituitary which then leads to ovulation. There is some evidence that a similar process can occur in some women for there are a number of reasonably well-documented cases where a single act of intercourse occurring just after or just before menstruation has been followed by pregnancy.

The menstrual cycle

The ovarian cycle of changing rates of hormone secretion is followed by cyclic changes in other organs produced by the hormones. The most obvious changes occur in the uterus, resulting in the menstrual cycle. Most of the features of the menstrual cycle can be imitated in women whose ovaries have been removed by giving a course of oestrogen alone for about two weeks, followed by oestrogen + progesterone for about 8–10 days and then by 5 days without hormones before the next oestrogen treatment begins.

The wall of the uterus is made up mainly of smooth muscle fibres and the cavity is lined by a special layer of tissue known as the endometrium. The endometrium is made of connective tissue. Its surface is covered by a ciliated epithelium and from the surface mucus-secreting glands dip down, into the apparently structureless connective tissue which is known as the stroma. There are two sorts of arteries, simple straight ones supply the deepest layers of the endometrium which are not shed during menstruation, while tortuous spiral vessels supply the more superficial layers.

At the end of menstruation, all the superficial layers are shed. The first stage in rebuilding is a rapid re-covering of the raw surface with ciliated epithelium. The glands at this stage are simple and

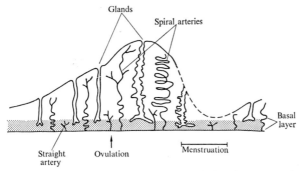

Fig.9.6. Changes in the endometrium which occur during the menstrual cycle.

straight. During the first half of the cycle (the follicular phase) the endometrium thickens slowly, the spiral arteries develop and the deepest parts of the glands become dilated. These effects are due to oestrogen and can be imitated by giving oestrogens to women without ovaries: on stopping the oestrogen treatment the endometrium breaks down and bleeding occurs but it is much less profuse than in a normal menstrual cycle.

During the luteal phase the thickening of the endometrium becomes much more rapid. The spiral arteries become tortuous and swollen with blood and the glands elongate rapidly becoming twisted and folded. These changes can be imitated in women without ovaries by following a course of oestrogen alone, with one of oestrogen + progestin. On cessation of the hormone treatment, bleeding occurs but this time is indistinguishable from that of a normal period. These observations suggest that menstrual bleeding is naturally due to a fall in the blood levels of oestrogen and progesterone at the end of the menstrual cycle.

Other organs apart from the uterus are also affected by the ovarian hormones. The cervical canal which leads from the uterus to the vagina has walls which secrete mucus. Increasing oestrogen concentrations make the mucus thinner, more alkaline and more easily penetrated by sperm. It is thinnest at the time of ovulation. Rising progesterone levels make the mucus thick, acid and difficult to penetrate. Cyclic changes also occur in the vaginal secretions but these are much less marked in humans than in many animals.

Just before menstruation many women become tense and irritable, concentrate less effectively and work less efficiently. The breasts enlarge and the tissues become loaded with salt and water. The reason for this 'premenstrual tension' is unknown, although it is almost certainly caused by fluctuating hormone levels of some sort.

SEXUAL INTERCOURSE

Sexual intercourse is a complex series of events which requires the interaction of two individuals. Variations in pattern are almost infinite and only the most basic physiological details will be described here.

The first problem which must be overcome is the deposition of sperm within the female genital tract. The penis in its normal flaccid state is a useless instrument for this purpose and so it must be converted into a stiff rod. This can be achieved because of the presence within the penis of three columns of spongy tissue, the corpora cavernosum. These are normally soft and relatively empty of blood. However, sexual excitement and particularly mechanical stimulation of the under side of the tip of the penis (the glans which is Latin for acorn) sets off the reflex. Parasympathetic nerves to the penile arteries release acetyl choline which makes them open wide. Sympathetic nerves to the penile arterioles are inhibited and this allows the arterioles also to dilate. Blood at high pressure can therefore be pumped into the corpora cavernosa. The venous outflow is simultaneously compressed and so the penis becomes hard and stiff as it fills with blood.

During normal sexual play before intercourse, corresponding changes take place in the female, again brought about by reflexes initiated by sexual excitement and by mechanical stimulation of the breasts and genitalia. The most important feature in the female is a rapid increase in the flow from the vagina of a lubricating mucus-rich solution: this allows the penis to slip easily into the vagina. The clitoris and labia also becomes congested with blood and the nipples stand erect.

When both partners are ready, the erect penis is slipped into the lubricated vagina. During movements of the penis in and out, the frictional stimuli in both partners should ideally result in simultaneous orgasm. In practice, male orgasm virtually always occurs while a failure to reach female orgasm is quite common.

In the male, orgasm results in the ejaculation of sperm from the tip of the penis. This occurs because the smooth muscle in the epididymis, the vas deferens, the prostate gland and the seminal vesicles all contract. Sperm are stored in the epididymis and vas and not in the seminal vesicles. The function of the vesicles is to secrete a fluid rich in fructose which bathes the sperm and supplies them with energy. The prostate gland secretes a complex fluid whose function is uncertain. The mixture of sperm, seminal vesicle fluid and prostatic fluid is known as semen. The normal ejaculate is 2–5 ml in volume and contains about 100 million sperm/ml. Frequent ejaculation reduces both the volume and the sperm count. Fertility seems to fall off when the count goes below 60 million/ml and successful fertilization is unlikely if it is below 20 million/ml.

During orgasm and simultaneously with the contraction of the smooth muscle, the skeletal muscles of the pelvis and penis contract, so helping the expulsion of sperm. During intercourse the blood pressure and heart rate rise considerably and this may put some strain on the cerebral blood vessels, especially in older people. Some strokes caused by cerebral haemorrhage occur during sexual intercourse.

In females, orgasm is associated with uterine movements, probably stimulated by oxytocin released from the posterior pituitary gland. This is strongly suggested by the fact that orgasm in lactating women is commonly associated with ejection of milk from the breasts. The importance of these uterine movements is uncertain. They have been thought to be important in the transport of sperm but many women who never achieve orgasm obviously have no trouble in conceiving.

FERTILIZATION AND SPERM TRANSPORT

It is believed that fertilization normally takes place near the ovarian end of the Fallopian tube. The sperm therefore have a long way to travel from the vagina. In the vagina many may be killed because the vaginal secretions are often acid and this kills the sperm. The prostatic and alkaline seminal vesicle secretions are alkaline and tend to reduce the acidity. The cervix probably offers the most difficult barrier for the sperm to surmount and it is important that around the

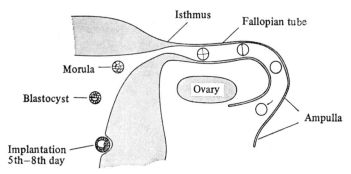

Fig.9.7. The female genital tract showing the probable site of fertilization and the stages the embryo goes through before implantation.

time of ovulation the cervical mucus should become thin. Once in the uterus, movements of the uterus and the Fallopian tubes, probably helped by cilia on the tube walls, assist the swimming sperm to reach their destination.

Fertilization occurs when a single sperm penetrates and fuses with the ovum to give the zygote. The zygote soon begins to divide, becoming first a solid mass of cells (morula) in which a cavity later appears (blastocyst). The journey down the tube to the uterus probably takes 2–5 days after which for several days, the embryo remains free in the uterine cavity. The outer layer of the embryo is known as the trophoblast and it is the trophoblast cells which burrow into the prepared endometrium and which stimulate the endometrium to form the maternal part of the placenta. This process is known as implantation.

PREGNANCY

The trophoblast of the implanted embryo differentiates into an outer layer where cell walls cannot be seen (syncytiotrophoblast) and an inner cellular layer (cytotrophoblast). Finger-like processes grow out from the trophoblast with blood vessels in their centres. These fetal blood vessels are connected to the main part of the fetus by the umbilical arteries and vein in the umbilical cord. On the maternal side of the placenta a cavity filled with blood develops into which the fetal villi project. Oxygen and food materials cross into the fetus from this lake while carbon dioxide and waste materials pass in the opposite direction.

Hormones during pregnancy

If fertilization occurs, the corpus luteum does not decay as in a usual cycle. Instead it continues to produce oestrogen and progesterone in order to maintain the uterine endometrium. How the ovary 'knows' that fertilization has taken place is one of the unsolved mysteries of the reproductive process. It may have something to do with a hormone called human chorionic gonadotrophin (HCG), which during the first three months is secreted by the placental trophoblast in enormous quantities. It is probably HCG which stimulates the corpus luteum to continue functioning. However, after 12–14 weeks of pregnancy the placenta itself secretes sufficient oestrogen and progesterone to maintain the pregnancy. The corpus luteum degenerates and, if necessary, the ovaries can be removed without terminating the pregnancy. If the ovaries are removed before three months abortion occurs.

The placenta is in fact an extremely important endocrine gland. The quantities of oestrogen and progesterone which it secretes increase steadily throughout pregnancy. In addition to these and to HCG it secretes two other hormones, making five in all:

1. Human placental lactogen (HPL). This has some of the properties of growth hormone and some of prolactin. It may be important in stimulating breast growth, in regulating metabolism, in relaxing smooth muscle and in regulating the renal excretion of sodium, potassium and water. It may be the hormone responsible for the retention in the body of salt and water which occurs during pregnancy.

2. Relaxin. This relaxes the ligaments which hold the pelvic joints and softens the soft tissues of the birth canal, so making it easier for the baby to pass along.

MATERNAL PHYSIOLOGY

During pregnancy many changes occur in the maternal organism which enable the mother to maintain the pregnancy and to be prepared for the tests of labour and lactation.

7

Cardiovascular system

The blood volume increases by about 30 per cent but the total red cell mass usually increases by less than this. As a result the red cell count and haemoglobin concentration tend to fall and this is so common that it has been called a 'physiological anaemia'. However, it has recently been shown that the anaemia may be partly due to folic acid and iron deficiencies, since if adequate supplements of both are given the increase in red cell mass tends to keep pace with the increase in blood volume. The cardiac output also increases to about 30–40 per cent above normal and does not fall until the baby has been delivered.

Smooth muscle in both arterioles and veins relaxes, possibly due to the combined effects of progesterone and HPL. There is a tendency for varicose veins to develop or to become worse partly because of smooth muscle relaxation and partly because the enlarging uterus impedes the return of blood from the lower limbs so tending to raise venous pressure.

Towards the end of pregnancy many women tend to faint if they lie on their backs. This is because the uterus presses on the inferior vena cava so preventing an adequate venous return of blood to the heart. If the blood cannot return it cannot be pumped out and so both cardiac output and blood pressure fall leading to fainting. This does not happen if a woman lies on her side.

Respiration

Breathing is stimulated, possibly by a direct action of progesterone on the brain. As a result the carbon dioxide level in the blood falls. The blood tends to become more alkaline and tetany (chapter 2) is not uncommon.

Alimentary tract

There is a general loss of smooth muscle tone which not uncommonly leads to constipation. In the early months of pregnancy there is often vomiting on getting up in the morning. The cause is unknown although it has been suggested that smooth muscle relaxation allows stomach fluid to pass back into the oesophagus where it leads to vomiting.

Urinary system

The blood flow to the kidneys and the glomerular filtration rate rise in parallel to the cardiac output. Many normal pregnant women have glucose in their urine, possibly because the increased filtration rate exceeds the reabsorptive capacity of the tubules. This finding does not mean that the woman is diabetic but may indicate the need for a glucose tolerance test.

The ureters share in the general loss of smooth muscle tone and become flaccid and dilated. The sphincters guarding the entrance to the bladder may become ineffective, so allowing urine (and infection) to pass backwards from the bladder up towards the kidneys.

Hormones

The blood levels of thyroid, parathyroid and adrenal cortical hormones all rise. Parathyroid hormone mobilizes bone calcium for transfer to the fetus. The high adrenal steroid levels may be responsible for the pigmented striae which often appear on the stretched abdomen and may also cause the remission of rheumatoid arthritis which sometimes occurs in pregnancy.

Weight

During a normal pregnancy the weight rises by 15–30 lb. About half of the rise can be attributed to the enlarging fetus, placenta and amniotic fluid volume. The other half is associated with increases in breast size, in blood volume, in interstitial fluid volume and in the deposition of body fat. There are very wide individual variations in the amount of weight put on and there is considerable argument about the mechanisms and meaning of the weight rise. Increased appetite may possibly be caused by progesterone and increased fluid retention by placental lactogen.

Pregnancy tests

These all depend on the fact that very early in pregnancy large amounts of HCG are excreted in the urine. HCG can cause ovulation in many species of animal and most of the tests used until relatively recently depended on the effects of injecting suspected pregnancy urine into mice, rabbits or toads. These biological tests have now been superseded by exceedingly efficient biochemical tests which do not use animals.

PARTURITION

During pregnancy there is an enormous growth of the uterus. Within 40 weeks it develops from a small organ deep within the pelvis to an enormous one which alters all intra-abdominal anatomy. Even in the non-pregnant state the uterus shows spontaneous contractions and this tendency of its muscle to contract is increased in pregnancy by two factors:

1. Stretching any form of smooth muscle tends to make it respond by contracting: uterine smooth muscle is no exception to this rule.

2. Oestrogens which are present in increasing concentrations as pregnancy progresses increase the power and excitability of the muscle.

What then prevents the uterus from contracting and expelling the infant long before the end of pregnancy? The answer is unknown, but two factors may be involved. Both progesterone and placental lactogen can inhibit uterine muscle activity. The levels of lactogen tend to fall during the last two weeks before parturition and progesterone levels also fall immediately before and during labour. This then leaves the factors which stimulate uterine muscle action with a free field.

During the course of pregnancy uterine activity goes through the following phases:

1. In early and mid-pregnancy it is very much depressed, even as compared to the non-pregnant level.

2. At about the time of the 30th week, spontaneous contractions begin and can be recorded by special techniques. These contractions do not involve a coordinated response of the whole uterine muscle and they are not painful.

3. During the last two weeks or so of the pregnancy, the mother becomes aware of irregular uterine contractions which gradually become stronger and more painful.

4. True labour begins when the contractions become coordinated and regular, recurring at 10–15 minute intervals. Normally the contractions start near the top (fundus) of the uterus and then sweep down and around the uterus pressing the infant's head against the cervix.

5. The fetal membranes rupture releasing the amniotic fluid which they contain and allowing the infant's head to press harder on the cervix. This pressure on the cervix activates sensory receptors: these receptors initiate a reflex which causes the release from the posterior pituitary gland of a hormone known as oxytocin, which is a powerful uterine stimulant. The contractions become more and more powerful

and closer and closer together in time so dilating the cervix and pushing the infant through and down into the vagina. At this stage the mother usually feels an irresistible urge to push downwards and to force the infant out.

6. Once the infant has been born, the placenta becomes detached from the wall of the uterus and is expelled: the uterus then contracts down over the raw surface to stop bleeding. Normally the expulsion of the placenta takes 30–60 minutes after birth of the infant but in most hospitals today, delivery of the placenta is accelerated by the injection at the time of delivery of the infant of a drug which strongly stimulates uterine contractions.

The mechanism which starts off the whole process of labour is unknown but recent work has suggested that the fetal pituitary and adrenal are important. In human infants or in animals whose pituitaries or adrenals are absent for some reason, pregnancy is almost always unduly prolonged. In experiments with sheep it has been demonstrated that this type of prolonged pregnancy can be quickly terminated by injecting cortisol through the abdominal wall into the *fetus*. Injection of cortisol into the mother has no effect. This suggests that the fetal pituitary at the appropriate time stimulates the fetal adrenals to secrete cortisol or a related hormone which then in an unknown way triggers off labour. A great deal of research remains to be carried out on this topic.

LACTATION

The process of lactation has three components:

1. The growth of the breasts from the non-pregnant state.
2. The synthesis and secretion of milk.
3. The ejection of the stored milk from the nipple.

The non-pregnant breast consists of some 15-25 lobes, each with a main duct which dilates and empties into collecting spaces beneath the pigmented area around the nipple (areola). Each main duct has many secondary ducts branching off it: these secondary ducts end in groups of secretory cells known as alveoli. Before pregnancy the ducts have few branches, the secretory cells are small and few in number and much of the breast is filled with fat. Oestrogen injections cause proliferation of the ducts, while oestrogen and progesterone together stimulate growth of the alveoli as well. Placental lactogen,

8

thyroid hormone and adrenal steroids are also all necessary for normal breast growth during pregnancy.

The breasts become capable of secreting milk at any time after about the fourth month of pregnancy but virtually no milk is secreted until after parturition. This is probably because the process of secretion is blocked by the high levels of progesterone present during pregnancy. At birth progesterone levels in the blood fall sharply as the placenta is expelled. The levels of placental lactogen also fall but prolactin from the anterior pituitary takes over its function of breast stimulation. The first fluid to be secreted is the watery, protein-rich, lipid-poor colostrum but within a few days

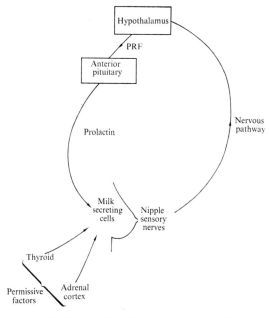

Fig.9.8. The control of milk secretion. Hormones from the thyroid and adrenal cortex (so-called 'permissive' factors) although they do not take part in the reflex itself are essential for the normal secretion of milk.

normal milk is secreted at a high rate. The colostrum contains maternal antibodies which at this early stage in the infant's life can be absorbed from the gut and may help to give the child some immunity to disease during its early months.

The secretion of milk depends on a reflex in which both nerves and hormones are involved. Suckling stimulates the nerves in the nipple and impulses travel up to the hypothalamus. The hypothalamus then alters the output of a factor which travels down the pituitary portal blood vessels and controls the output of prolactin. So long as suckling continues, a high rate of prolactin secretion is maintained. When suckling stops the secretion of prolactin falls and the secretion of milk soon stops.

The ejection of the secreted milk from the breast also depends on the interaction of nerves and hormones. Again the process begins with suckling which activates nipple sensory nerves. Again the impulses ascend to the hypothalamus. But this time the hypothalamus

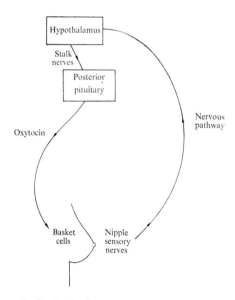

Fig.9.9. The control of milk ejection.

sends impulses down to the posterior pituitary where oxytocin is released. The oxytocin then circulates in the blood back to the breasts. Surrounding the ducts of the breasts are special cells known as myo-epithelial cells which contract in response to oxytocin, so pushing the milk out. The hormonal part of the mechanism explains why the milk does not flow freely until a minute or two after suckling starts.

CONTRACEPTION

The only permanent answer to the population explosion lies in the increased availability and use of contraception. Broadly speaking, contraceptive techniques may be divided into those which require strong motivation, moderate intelligence and forethought before intercourse and those which do not require these factors. The main methods in use are as follows:

1. Coitus interruptus, or withdrawal of the penis just before male orgasm. This method is unsatisfactory and very frequently ineffective.

2. The rhythm method, which depends on the fact that in women with regular cycles, ovulation rarely occurs outside the 9th and 19th days after the beginning of the menstrual bleed. Intercourse is avoided during the ten day interval. This method is ineffective in women who do not have regular cycles and requires very considerable self control by the partners.

3. The rubber diaphragm which fits into the vagina over the cervix and which is often combined with the use in the vagina of spermicidal jelly or foam. This method is effective when the diaphragm is fitted properly.

4. The condom or sheath which is fitted on to the erect penis and which catches the sperm and stops them entering the vagina.

5. Oral contraceptives, which seem to depend on the suppression of LH secretion and thus of ovulation by means of combinations of oestrogens and progestins. A pill is taken every day for three weeks and then withdrawn for a week during which an artificial, scanty menstrual bleed occurs. The method is 100 per cent effective and is popular because it requires no thought or action before intercourse. It does cause depression, weight gain, high blood pressure and other changes in a relatively small proportion of users. In a tiny fraction of women it may cause clotting of the blood and any woman with a known tendency to abnormal clotting should not use the pill. In most countries the dangers of taking the pill are considerably less than the dangers of pregnancy.

6. Progestin implants which release a small amount of progestin daily and which can prevent conception for many months. The mode of action is uncertain but may be partly due to an action on ovulation and partly due to an effect on the uterus or Fallopian tubes.

7. The intra-uterine device (IUD or 'coil') which stops pregnancy by an unknown mechanism, possibly by interfering with implantation. A small plastic device is introduced into the uterine cavity and remains there until pregnancy is desired: it is only a little less effective than the pill. In a proportion of women it causes unpleasant side effects such as painful periods and it is rarely used in those who have not borne children.

8. Sterilization. Tying of the Fallopian tubes in women or the vasa in men leads to sterility. The female operation requires a general anaesthetic and abdominal incision while the male one can be done in a few minutes under local anaesthesia. The method is highly reliable but for obvious reasons is normally carried out only on those who have had at least two or three children. Considerable research is being carried out into techniques which will allow the operation to be reversible.

9. Abortion. This can be effective but surgical abortion can be carried out on a large scale only in highly developed countries where the hospitals, staff and finance are available. Surgical abortion used routinely as a method of controlling population leads to many ethical problems. It seems possible that in the future, however, the place of abortion may be revolutionized by the widespread use of substances known as prostaglandins which were first isolated from prostatic fluid. They are very powerful stimulators of uterine muscle and in some centres the intravenous infusion of prostaglandin is used routinely for inducing abortion. The aim however is to produce either a pill or a vaginal pessary which contains prostaglandins and which can be used to stimulate uterine contractions and menstruation in any woman whose period is a few days overdue. The hope is that such medication may be able to be administered by the patient herself which would virtually eliminate the need for surgical abortion.

10

The fetus and child

The development of the fetus goes through two main stages. During the first ten weeks or so all the major organ systems of the body are formed. From about the 10th week to term, all the organs grow and mature but there are few new major developments. Most important congenital abnormalities are determined by the 10th week of pregnancy and this is why it is particularly important to avoid exposure to rubella (German measles) and possibly harmful drugs during the first three months of pregnancy.

In a human being outside the uterus, lungs, gut and kidneys are all vital. But in the fetus the functions of these organs, providing food and oxygen and eliminating carbon dioxide and waste, are all carried out by the mother operating through the placenta. It is therefore not surprising that embryos with major defects in gut, lung and kidneys can survive until they are born at the normal time.

As well as allowing essential substances to pass easily, the placenta forms a very effective barrier to many factors which could harm the fetus. Bacteria cannot normally cross the placenta: the only major exception to this rule is syphilis and thus syphilis in the mother is almost always passed on to the child. Protozoa too do not normally cross the placenta, the main exception being toxoplasma which is very common throughout the world. In adults, infection with toxoplasma (toxoplasmosis) is normally symptomless but in the fetus it may cause severe damage, especially to the brain. As might be expected from their small size, a number of viruses can cross the placenta. The best known of these is rubella but there are a number of others including the viruses which cause hepatitis.

The maternal and fetal circulations do not come into actual contact since they are separated by the trophoblast. However, during the violent uterine contractions which occur during parturition, it is almost inevitable that some fetal blood will enter the mother. This can of course lead to problems in later pregnancies if the mother is Rh— and the fetus is Rh+ (chapter 4).

Another problem is that the fetus is immunologically different from the mother and therefore ought to be rejected by the mother like a foreign kidney or heart graft. Some theories of the beginning of labour have been based on the rejection idea. However it has now been demonstrated that the fetal trophoblast is covered by an immunologically inert layer, rich in sialic and hyaluronic acids. This layer keeps maternal and fetal tissues safely apart and prevents rejection.

FETAL CARDIOVASCULAR SYSTEM

In the fetus the cardiovascular system is the most important system of all, since survival depends on the blood being pumped out along the umbilical cord to the placenta and back again. Fetal blood has a higher affinity for oxygen than adult blood: it contains a special type of haemoglobin, HbF, which has a very strong attraction for oxygen. HbF has virtually disappeared from the infant's blood within four months after birth.

The important features of the fetal circulation are shown in Fig.10.1 The main points to note are:

1. Oxygenated blood returns from the placenta via the umbilical vein. Most passes via the ductus venosus directly to the inferior vena cava where it is mixed with blood from the lower limbs. The rest goes to the left two thirds of the liver and enters the vena cava via the hepatic veins. The right one third of the liver is supplied by the portal vein.

2. Two streams of blood enter the right atrium. These are a partially oxygenated stream from the inferior vena cava and a deoxygenated stream from the superior vena cava. It has been shown that these two streams mix very little. The oxygenated blood flows straight through the foramen ovale into the left atrium while the deoxygenated stream passes to the right ventricle and is pumped out along the pulmonary artery.

3. Some of the pulmonary artery blood enters the pulmonary circulation and returns to the left atrium but most passes across into the descending aorta by way of the ductus arteriosus.

4. The oxygenated blood is pumped into the aorta by the left ventricle and enters the carotid and subclavian arteries.

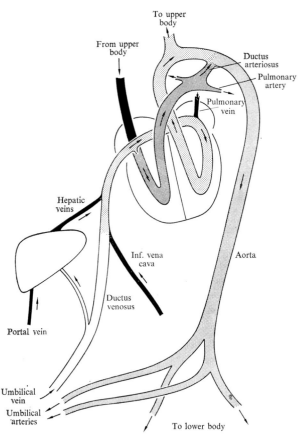

Fig.10.1. The fetal circulation. The degree of shading gives a rough indication of the level of oxygenation, light indicating oxygenated and dark deoxygenated blood.

5. Some of the blood in the descending aorta supplies the lower limbs and body but most passes via the paired umbilical arteries to the placenta.

THE SHOCK OF BIRTH

When the fetus emerges from the mother the umbilical cord is clamped and divided by the doctor or midwife so cutting off irrevocably the infant from the placenta. Even if the cord were not cut, on exposure to the outside air the umbilical vessels would contract and close as happens, of course, in animals. There is increasing evidence that immediate clamping of the cord before its natural pulsations have ceased may actually be harmful and may be a cause of anaemia in the new-born infant. Quite large amounts of fetal blood are present in the placenta and in the absence of inter-ference uterine contractions force this blood along the umbilical cord into the infant. It is therefore sensible to wait for a few moments before clamping and tying the cord.

The immediate problem which faces the new-born child is that of supplying oxygen to its body. In the fetus, the lungs are functionless and they receive very little blood: most of the blood which enters the pulmonary artery is transferred directly to the aorta via the ductus arteriosus. In the new born infant, in contrast, the lungs are vital and must quickly expand while the pulmonary artery must carry to the lungs as much blood as the aorta carries to the rest of the body.

Respiration

In normal infants lung expansion presents few problems. Sensory stimuli resulting from the sudden emergence into the outside world initiate reflex breathing movements which automatically suck air into the chest. A few infants actually cry and breathe when only the head has emerged from the vagina and while the umbilical cord is still intact: in these cases only sensory stimuli from the head region must be required to initiate breathing. Other infants do not breathe until the cord has stopped pulsating or has been clamped and the oxygenation of the fetal blood falls. The least vigorous infants may give only ineffective gasps or may fail to breathe at all. Maternal anaesthesia and analgesia and long and difficult labours in which the cord may be compressed and the oxygen supply to the fetus reduced long before birth actually takes place are all associated with trouble in initiating breathing. In these cases slapping, cold or warm water on the skin, distension of the anal sphincter and (most important of all) cautious artificial ventilation with an oxygen-rich mixture may start respiration. The force that must be applied to expand the lungs in the first breaths is very large and in the absence of alveolar detergent (chapter 6) lung expansion may be impossible and the infant may die of the respiratory distress syndrome.

Circulation

Changes in the circulation are just as important as and are comple-mentary to the changes in the lungs. The main features are:

1. When the umbilical cord closes down there is a sharp increase in the resistance to the outflow of the left ventricle. As a consequence, the blood pressures in the aorta, left ventricle and left atrium all tend to rise.

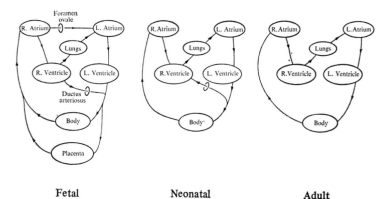

Fetal   Neonatal   Adult

Fig.10.2. Outlines of the circulation in the fetus, new-born infant and adult.

2. The closing of the cord cuts off the venous return from the placenta and reduces the inflow of blood to the right side of the heart. Pressures in the right atrium, right ventricle and pulmonary artery all fall.

3. Expansion of the lungs greatly reduces the resistance to blood flow through them. This lowering of pulmonary resistance tends to lower blood pressure in the pulmonary artery, right ventricle and right atrium.

4. Because of these changes, pressure in the right atrium becomes lower than that in the left atrium. As a result the foramen ovale closes with a valve-like action and soon becomes permanently sealed.

5. Because the pressure in the aorta becomes higher than that in the pulmonary artery, the direction of blood flow through the ductus arteriosus changes. It flows from aorta to pulmonary artery instead of in the reverse direction. This means that the blood from the aorta goes round to the lungs again for a second helping of oxygen. When the oxygen saturation of the blood flowing through the ductus reaches about 90 per cent, the ductus closes and the adult form of circulation becomes operative.

THE NEW-BORN INFANT

Once the infant has overcome the immediate shock of adjusting its respiratory and cardiovascular systems to the demands of the outside world it is faced with further problems.

The gut

At birth the gut is filled with a substance known as meconium which consists of partially digested epithelial cells which have been shed from the gut wall and which is usually stained green with biliverdin, a breakdown product of bile. The stools are therefore at first green. Within a few days they become brownish-yellow. This is an important sign because it indicates that new faeces are being formed from milk products and that the gut must therefore be open along its whole length. Many congenital abnormalities can cause partial or complete blockage of the gut.

During the first few days of life all infants lose weight, partly because of inadequate water intake and partly because the nutritive value of maternal milk may be poor at this time. Most milk diets are deficient in iron and so until it is weaned the infant must survive on its own iron stores built up during the last part of intra-uterine life.

Temperature regulation

Body temperature in infants is unstable. This is primarily because methods of controlling heat loss using the skin circulation and sweat glands are not well developed. The shivering mechanism is also ineffective in infants. It is therefore very important to keep new-born infants warm.

Liver

The liver contains large stores of glycogen at birth but within a few hours the glycogen is used up by conversion to glucose and the blood glucose level falls. The fall in blood glucose is particularly severe in small and premature infants and if untreated it can cause brain damage or even death. It is therefore important to check on the blood glucose concentration in infants who are at risk.

In the fetus, bilirubin resulting from haemoglobin breakdown is for the most part disposed of across the placenta. After birth, before bilirubin can be excreted into the gut, it must be conjugated with glucuronic acid by the liver (Table 10.1.). During the first week of life the mechanisms for carrying out this reaction are poorly developed. Free bilirubin therefore tends to accumulate in the liver blood and may cause jaundice. This is unlikely to be dangerous in a normal infant but in premature babies and in those in whom haemolysis is excessive because of rhesus disease, dangerously high levels of bilirubin may occur and can cause brain damage (kernicterus).

Table 10.1. The metabolism of the bile pigments

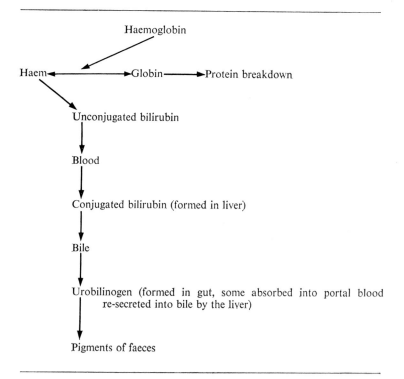

Haemoglobin

Haem ← Globin → Protein breakdown

Unconjugated bilirubin

Blood

Conjugated bilirubin (formed in liver)

Bile

Urobilinogen (formed in gut, some absorbed into portal blood re-secreted into bile by the liver)

Pigments of faeces

CHILDHOOD

The most obvious physical features of childhood are growth in height and weight. The tissues of the body can be divided into four groups according to the growth curve which they follow (Fig.10.3.).

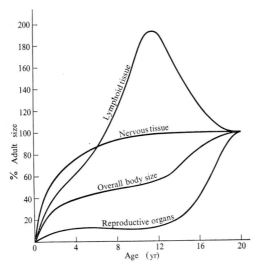

Fig.10.3. Patterns of growth of different tissues, their size being expressed as a percentage of their size in the adult.

With the exception of the reproductive organs, all tissues grow rapidly after birth. Rapid growth of nervous tissue continues until the age of 8–9 when it has almost reached the final adult mass. Lymphoid tissue has an unusual pattern reaching very high levels around puberty and then falling to the final adult mass during the 'teen' years. The reproductive organs grow little until puberty when there is a sudden spurt. There are also changes in overall body shape (Fig.10.4.). The decreasing relative size of the head is a reflection of the early growth of nervous tissue.

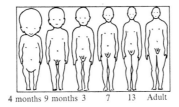

4 months 9 months 3   7   13   Adult

Fig.10.4. The changes in male body shape and contour which take place during life.

The maximal height to which an individual can grow is probably genetically determined but many other factors decide whether the maximal height will be reached. Nutrition is the most important of these and malnutrition is a major cause of poor physical development. Normal growth seems to require the interaction of growth hormone from the pituitary, the adrenal hormones and thyroid hormone.

PUBERTY

Puberty is the period of life when the gonads grow rapidly, when the output of sex hormones leads to the development of secondary sexual characters and when mature ova or sperm are released for the first time. The main features of puberty were described in the last chapter. In girls the first signs are pubic hair growth and breast development: they precede menarche by 1–2 years. In boys growth of pubic hair and the penis are the first signs. In girls the first signs of puberty tend to occur 1–2 years earlier than in boys but there is wide individual variation. For example about 5 per cent of normal girls show some sign of puberty at the age of 10 while about 5 per cent of normal boys show no signs until they are 15.

Before puberty there is relatively little difference between the heights and weights of girls and boys. Boys tend to be a little taller during infancy and very early childhood, while between the ages of 8 and 13 girls may become taller and heavier because they show an earlier pubertal growth spurt. This spurt is usually before the menarche and relatively little growth occurs afterwards. Boys eventually become taller and heavier than girls because they have a longer pre-pubertal growth period and the pubertal spurt is greater. Adrenal androgens are probably very important in causing growth at the time of puberty.

11

Responses
of the whole body

Up until this chapter we have been primarily concerned with discussing the behaviour of individual systems in the body. This is clearly an over-simplified and artificial way of looking at things for in the normal individual all the systems work closely together for the good of the whole. In this chapter we shall be considering various situations in which the physiology must be considered in terms of the responses of the whole body.

TEMPERATURE REGULATION

Everyone knows that the 'body' has a 'steady temperature' but not many know precisely what the terms 'body' and 'steady temperature' mean. The parts of the body whose temperature is most closely regulated are the arterial blood and the brain. Yet even these tissues do not have a temperature which is absolutely steady at 98·6 °F or 37 °C. There is considerable variation during the day. In most people the daily variation in temperature is around 1 °F but in some entirely normal individuals it may be as much as 2 °F. Temperatures are lowest in the early morning and highest in the early evening, a normal variation of from 97 °F to 99 °F being not unknown. A minor degree of apparent temperature elevation early in the evening is therefore not necessarily pathological.

As well as variation of body temperature with time, there is also variation between different parts of the body. Most of the deep organs closely reflect the temperature of arterial blood but working muscles and the highly active liver may be 1–2 °F higher than the blood. Skin temperature varies enormously. It is usually much colder than that of arterial blood but in hot climates when the skin blood vessels are open wide in order to lose heat, the skin temperature may be close to that of arterial blood.

Arterial blood temperature is normally measured indirectly by thermometers placed in the mouth, axilla or rectum: the thermometer should usually be left in position for two minutes if an accurate reading is to be obtained. Of the three sites the temperature of the mouth most closely reflects that of arterial blood. The temperature of the axilla tends to be a little lower and that of the rectum a little higher. With infants it is easiest to take their temperatures by means of a rectal thermometer.

The reason for the need to maintain a relatively steady body temperature is that many of the basic biochemical and physical processes which go on in the body are temperature dependent. In general, heat tends to speed them up and cold to slow them down, although if the heat is sufficient to damage protein molecules then heat may cause destruction of cells. The behaviour of enzymes and of the nervous system are particularly temperature dependent. One of the main features of either too high a temperature or too low a temperature is disordered brain function, with the delirium of fever or the sluggishness and coma of hypothermia (low temperature).

Control of heat production

As a result of its metabolic activities the body continually produces heat. The amount of heat output in a given time in someone who is truly at rest and who has not eaten for at least 12 hours is known as the basal metabolic rate (BMR). There are four main ways in which the amount of heat produced by the body may be increased:

1. By voluntary exercise.

2. By the form of involuntary exercise known as shivering.

3. By increasing the rate of secretion of adrenaline (epinephrine) from the adrenal medulla. This breaks down glycogen in liver and muscle and increases the metabolic rate by increasing the availability of glucose.

4. By increasing the output of thyroid hormone which raises the basal metabolic rate. This seems to be a long term response which occurs in those exposed to cold for prolonged periods but it does not seem to operate in the short term.

Control of heat loss

The rate of transfer of heat from the body to the outside world depends on the following factors:

1. The temperature gradient between the body and its surroundings. If the environmental temperature is very low, heat will be lost rapidly. In a few parts of the world during the day time the environmental temperature may be above body temperature and so the body may actually gain heat from its surroundings.

2. The amount of body surface exposed and the effectiveness of the insulation of the body coverings. Heat is lost or gained most easily across bare skin and the amount of heat transfer decreases as the effectiveness of the insulation provided by clothing increases.

The main ways in which the body can regulate the rate of heat loss are as follows:

1. By changing behaviour. Heat loss will clearly be more effective in a cool environment than in a hot one. It is therefore possible to increase the rate of heat loss by moving to a cool place and seeking shade. Only 'mad dogs and Englishmen go out in the mid-day sun'.

2. By altering the amount of clothing worn.

3. By altering the amount of blood flowing through the skin. Skin blood flow is extremely variable. When all the skin vessels are opened up, the skin is as warm as arterial blood and heat loss from the body will be made easier. When all the skin vessels are closed down, skin temperature will become similar to that of the environment and there will therefore be minimal heat transfer between the skin and its surroundings. When the skin vessels are closed down, there is then a layer of insulating fat between the deep parts of the body and skin.

4. By altering the rate of sweating. Sweating is an effective way of losing heat because when 1 ml of water evaporates, it takes about 540 calories from its surroundings. This heat is known as latent heat and it means that when water evaporates from the skin, the skin will be cooled. Evaporation and therefore heat loss can occur even in situations when the surrounding environment is hotter than the body itself. However, the ease with which water evaporates depends on the relative humidity of the air. If the relative humidity is 100 per cent this means that the air is carrying all the water vapour that it can and no more can evaporate. Sweating will therefore be an ineffective method of heat loss and the sweat will run off the skin without

evaporating. This explains why hot, humid, 'sticky' environments such as the West Coast of Africa or the Mississippi Valley of the USA are so uncomfortable. In contrast, if the relative humidity is low, as in deserts, evaporation is rapid and sweating is a very effective way of losing heat. This is why desert climates are often relatively pleasant even though the actual environmental temperature may be very high.

The temperature control system

Like all control systems, the one which regulates temperature has three basic components, receptors, a central control mechanism and effectors. We have already discussed the effectors, the mechanisms

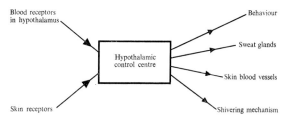

Fig.11.1. The temperature control system.

for regulating heat production and heat loss. Where are the receptors and the control centre? There are two sets of receptors:

1. Receptors in the skin which measure the temperature of the environment. Everyone is aware of the functioning of these receptors. They are important in producing modifications of behaviour and in warning the control centre of changes in the environment which may lead to changes in the temperature of the body.

2. Receptors in the brain (hypothalamus) which measure the temperature of the arterial blood itself.

The central control mechanism is also in the hypothalamus. It receives information from all the receptors and in accordance with this it modifies the behaviour of the effectors. If the body temperature is too high, heat production is cut down by reducing muscular activity and heat loss is increased by seeking a cool environment, by sweating and by increasing the blood flow to the skin. If the body temperature is too low, heat production may be increased by exercise, shivering or adrenaline, while heat loss may be cut down by reducing skin blood flow. The skin, especially in the extremities, becomes cold and often blue due to deoxygenation of the sluggishly flowing blood.

Fever

The commonest abnormality of temperature regulation is fever, the elevation of temperature which occurs in inflammatory disease of any sort whether due to infection, tissue damage because of injury, or cancer. The function of fever is unknown: it does not appear to enhance the body's ability to cope with disease. The only common organism which may be killed by the temperatures reached in fever is the spirochaete of syphilis. Unfortunately syphilis itself does not produce fever of sufficient degree to kill the spirochaetes. However, if someone with syphilis becomes infected with malaria, the high temperatures reached because of the malaria will kill the spirochaetes. Before the development of modern chemotherapy it was therefore not uncommon to treat syphilis by causing a deliberate malarial infection.

In fever the central regulating mechanism is reset so that it operates around a new temperature. Instead of regarding, say, 98·6 °F as the normal body temperature, the control centre comes to regard, say 104 °F, as 'normal'. A truly normal temperature is therefore far too low as far as the hypothalamic control centre is concerned. The control centre therefore orders an increase in heat production by shivering and a reduction in heat loss by means of constriction of skin blood vessels: the patient feels cold. As a result of these effector actions the body temperature rises until it reaches 104 °F and the hypothalamus regulates around this new level. At the termination of the fever the hypothalamus again comes to regard a temperature of, say 98·6 °F, as normal. 104 °F is obviously far too high and the temperature is rapidly brought down by sweating and an increase in blood flow to the skin.

The change in behaviour of the hypothalamus in fever seems to be brought about by substances called pyrogens which are high molecular weight carbohydrates. Pyrogens are released by leucocytes which become involved in an inflammatory reaction and circulate in the blood to act on the brain.

Menstrual cycle

Women show variations of the early morning arterial temperature during the menstrual cycle. Body temperature is at a minimum at the time of menstruation, rises slowly during the first half of the cycle and then shows a sharp jump of about 0·5 °C at the time of ovulation. The increase is probably due to action on metabolism of progesterone which is secreted at about this time. The rise in temperature can be used to indicate ovulation both in women desiring conception and in those trying to avoid it.

Heat stress

People who live in hot environments may show a number of different types of illness associated with the problem of keeping cool.

1. Cramps. Those who work in a hot and humid environment often suffer cramps. These occur because sweat contains salt as well as water and so at high rate of sweating there is considerable salt loss. Loss of sweat tends to be replaced by the drinking of water only: the body therefore becomes salt depleted and cramps result. The condition may be cured by drinking dilute salt solutions for fluid replacement or by taking ample salt with meals.

2. Prickly heat. During periods of prolonged sweating, the superficial layers of the skin may become soft and block the ducts of the sweat glands. Sweat therefore cannot escape and produces little pustules which are extremely itchy and very easily become infected.

3. Heat exhaustion and heat stroke. These occur when fluid is lost by sweating and not replaced. First there is a feeling of light headedness and weakness which may progress to weakness nausea and vomiting. Up to this stage body temperature is usually little above normal and the patient recovers quickly if given adequate fluids and salt by mouth: this stage is often known as heat exhaustion. However, if the sweat loss continues further without replacement, a stage may eventually be reached when the body water is so depleted that sweating stops and the blood becomes very viscous ('sticky') because of the water loss. When sweating stops, the body temperature begins to rise rapidly and if nothing is done death will occur soon, preceded by delirium and then unconsciousness. This stage is known as heat stroke and requires urgent treatment. The patient must be cooled as quickly as possible by being bathed in iced water. At the same time fluids and electrolytes must be replaced intravenously and the limbs must be vigorously massaged to increase skin blood flow and heat loss.

EXERCISE

Exercise is another excellent example of the interaction of several systems of the body to produce a coordinated response. Exercise begins when the central nervous system sends instructions to the muscles to begin working. The muscles move the joints and a whole complex series of events is initiated.

Respiration

When exercise occurs, four sensory stimuli may increase the rate of breathing:

1. Receptors in the joints inform the respiratory control centre that exercise is occurring and that the breathing rate must be faster if oxygen is going to be supplied and carbon dioxide is going to be removed fast enough.

2. The exercising muscles produce carbon dioxide more rapidly than usual. This tends to raise the carbon dioxide level in arterial blood and stimulates the chemoreceptors in the carotid and aortic bodies and the medulla oblongata. As a result of the information the control centre raises the respiration rate until the rate of carbon dioxide loss elimination keeps pace with its production and the arterial partial pressure of carbon dioxide is brought back to normal.

3. Exercising muscles may produce acids such as lactic acid which may also stimulate chemoreceptors.

4. Exercising muscles use up oxygen and the tendency for oxygen levels to fall may stimulate the chemoreceptors, although in normal circumstances carbon dioxide excess is a more important stimulus than oxygen lack.

As a result of all these stimuli, the ventilation rate may increase tenfold, greatly increasing the rate of oxygen supply and carbon dioxide removal.

Cardiovascular system

It would not be of much use to supply more oxygen by increasing the ventilation rate if the cardiac output were not increased to supply the oxygen rapidly to the working muscles. The cardiac output may rise from 4–5 litres/min at rest to over 35 litres/min in very severe exercise. The rise in cardiac output is brought about partly by an increase in heart rate and partly by an increase in stroke volume. The heart muscle contracts more vigorously and with each beat pumps out a greater proportion of the blood it contains. Sympathetic nerves to the heart and adrenaline released from the adrenal medulla are important in stimulating the heart to beat more rapidly and more vigorously.

Not only does the cardiac output increase but the distribution of blood to the various organs changes. Arterioles in the muscles open wide, partly because of reduction of sympathetic activity but more because of the local effects of high carbon dioxide and reduced oxygen levels. This dilatation results in a large increase in muscle blood flow. Part of the demand is met by the increase in cardiac output and part by a reduction of flow to the gut and kidneys to about one fifth of the normal rate or even less. This is why it is unwise to do strenuous exercise immediately after a meal: blood is diverted from the gut and digestion does not take place satisfactorily.

The blood flow to the skin is important in exercise because it offers a way of getting rid of the extra heat produced by muscular activity. The skin blood vessels open wide giving a warm, red skin. Sweating is usually profuse. If the rate of heat elimination were not greatly increased during exercise the body temperature could rise rapidly and dangerously: as it is a rise of 2–3 °F is not uncommon.

Metabolism

One of the major problems in exercise is to provide fuel for energy to the working muscles, while simultaneously not allowing the muscles to take so much glucose from the blood that the energy supply to the brain is put in danger. This is achieved primarily by the actions of adrenaline released from the adrenal medulla. This acts in the following ways:

1. It stimulates the breakdown of glycogen stored within the muscles so increasing the supply of glucose within the muscle fibres.

2. It stimulates the breakdown of liver glycogen to glucose. This glucose enters the blood and helps to maintain normal levels.

3. It reduces the rate at which the muscles take glucose from the blood.

By these actions adrenaline increases the internal energy supply to the muscles, while simultaneously preventing a sharp fall of blood glucose which might endanger brain blood supply.

The oxygen supply in exercise, even though it is increased enormously often cannot keep pace with the oxygen requirements of the muscles. As a result lactic acid, which is produced when oxygen supply is insufficient, accumulates. After the exercise is over the lactic acid can be converted by both muscle and liver first into pyruvic acid and then into glycogen. This process requires oxygen and so the consumption of oxygen remains relatively high even after the exercise has finished.

ACID-BASE BALANCE

There are two main problems in acid-base balance:

1. Considerable amounts of carbon dioxide enter the blood in the capillaries. When the body is in equilibrium, equal amounts of carbon dioxide are lost again in the lungs. Since carbon dioxide when dissolved in water gives rise first to carbonic acid (H_2CO_3) which then splits up to give H^+ and HCO_3^- ions, considerable amounts of hydrogen ions are added to the blood in the capillaries and then removed again in the lungs. It is desirable that the impact of these hydrogen ions on the pH of the blood should be minimized. This can be achieved because the buffer systems of the blood remove many of the hydrogen ions from solution. Haemoglobin is by far the most important of these buffers. When it gives up oxygen in the capillaries it becomes a weaker acid than when it is fully oxygenated. Weak acids take up hydrogen ions and so the haemoglobin combines with most of the hydrogen ions added to the blood by the carbon dioxide, thus keeping actual changes in pH to a minimum.

2. When the body is in equilibrium, the kidneys and the lungs eliminate precisely the same number of hydrogen ions per minute as are formed per minute. The lungs eliminate the hydrogen ions by getting rid of the gas, carbon dioxide, while the kidneys secrete hydrogen ions into the urine. This equilibrium can be upset in four major ways which are outlined in the remainder of this section.

Respiratory acidosis

This occurs when for some reason the lungs cannot get rid of carbon dioxide as quickly as they normally can. Respiratory diseases such as asthma are common causes of respiratory acidosis. The carbon dioxide accumulates in the arterial blood and makes it more acid. If the respiratory problem continues for some time, the pH of the blood may be brought back nearly to normal because the kidney secretes more hydrogen ions into the urine and at the same time secretes bicarbonate ions into the blood.

Respiratory alkalosis

This occurs when the lungs get rid of carbon dioxide more quickly than usual. As a consequence the carbon dioxide level in arterial blood falls and the blood becomes more alkaline. Respiratory alkalosis usually occurs during hysteria when the person mistakenly thinks that she is not breathing rapidly enough: she therefore tries to overbreathe and gets rid of too much carbon dioxide. The condition occurs during labour and also at high altitudes when the respiration may be driven by oxygen lack. In the latter situation in order to supply enough oxygen for the body's need it is essential to breathe more rapidly than is necessary for the elimination of carbon dioxide and so carbon dioxide levels fall. The main obvious consequence of respiratory alkalosis is tetany (chapter 2) which occurs because free calcium ions become bound by plasma proteins. Again if the excessive breathing continues for a long period, blood pH may be brought back towards normal because the kidney compensates by secreting less hydrogen ions and more bicarbonate ions.

Metabolic acidosis

This can occur when excessive amounts of hydrogen ions are produced as in diabetic coma or when the excretion of hydrogen ions by the kidneys fails as in renal failure. Either way the concentration of hydrogen ions in the blood rises. This time it is the respiratory system which attempts to compensate and to bring the blood pH back towards normal. The hydrogen ions stimulate the chemical receptors in the aortic and carotid bodies and this stimulation leads to an increased ventilation rate. The carbon dioxide level in the blood therefore falls and this tends to return blood pH back to normal.

Metabolic alkalosis

This occurs when excessive amounts of hydrogen ions are lost from the body. By far the commonest cause is vomiting of acid gastric juice. The loss of acid leaves the blood excessively alkaline. The alkalinity depresses the breathing and so more carbon dioxide tends to accumulate in the blood. The increasing amounts of carbon dioxide compensate for the lost hydrogen ions and return blood pH towards normal.

Index